KAREN HORNEY, M.D.

Our
Inner Conflicts

A CONSTRUCTIVE THEORY
OF NEUROSIS

W · W · NORTON & COMPANY · INC ·
NEW YORK

PRINTED IN THE UNITED STATES OF AMERICA
123456789

Contents

Preface

THIS BOOK is dedicated to the advancement of psychoanalysis. It has grown out of my experience in analytical
work with my patients and with myself. While the theory it presents evolved over a period of years, it was not
until I undertook the preparation of a series of lectures
under the auspices of the American Institute for Psychoanalysis that my ideas finally crystallized. The first
of these, centering about the technical aspects of the
subject, was entitled "Problems of Psychoanalytical
Technique" (1943). The second series, which covered
the problems dealt with here, was given in 1944 under
the title "Integration of Personality." Selected subjects
—"Integration of Personality in Psychoanalytical Therapy," "The Psychology of Detachment," and "The
Meaning of Sadistic Trends"—have been presented at
the Academy of Medicine and before the Association
for the Advancement of Psychoanalysis.

It is my hope that the book will be useful to psycho-
analysts who are seriously interested in improving our
theory and therapy. I hope also that they will not only
make the ideas presented here available to their patients
but will apply them to themselves as well. Progress in
psychoanalysis can only be made the hard way, by including ourselves and our difficulties. If we remain static
and averse to change, our theories are bound to become
barren and dogmatic.

I am convinced, however, that any book that goes beyond the range of merely technical matters or abstract psychological theory should benefit also all those who want to know themselves and have not given up struggling for their own growth. Most of us who live in this difficult civilization are caught in the conflicts described here and need all the help we can get. Though severe neuroses belong in the hands of experts, I still believe that with untiring effort we can ourselves go a long way toward disentangling our own conflicts.

My prime gratitude belongs to my patients who, in our work together, have given me a better understanding of neurosis. I am also indebted to my colleagues who have encouraged my work by their interest and sympathetic understanding. I refer not only to my older colleagues but also to the younger ones, trained in our Institute, whose critical discussions have been stimulating and fruitful.

I want to mention three persons outside the field of psychoanalysis who in their own particular ways have given me support in the furtherance of my work. It was Dr. Alvin Johnson who gave me the opportunity to present my ideas at the New School for Social Research at a time when classical Freudian analysis was the only recognized school of analytical theory and practice. More especially I am indebted to Clara Mayer, Dean of the School of Philosophy and Liberal Arts of the New School for Social Research. By her continued personal interest she has encouraged me, year after year, to offer for discussion whatever new findings were garnered from my analytical work. And then there is my publisher, W. W. Norton, whose helpful advice has led to many improvements in my books. Last but not least, I want to express my appreciation to Minette Kuhn who has helped me greatly toward a better organization of the material and a clearer formulation of my ideas.

K. H.

Introduction

WHATEVER the starting point and however tortuous the road, we must finally arrive at a disturbance of personality as the source of psychic illness. The same can be said of this as of almost any other psychological discovery: it is really a rediscovery. Poets and philosophers of all times have known that it is never the serene, well-balanced person who falls victim to psychic disorders, but the one torn by inner conflicts. In modern terms, every neurosis, no matter what the symptomatic picture, is a character neurosis. Hence our endeavor in theory and therapy must be directed toward a better understanding of the neurotic character structure.

Actually, Freud's great pioneering work increasingly converged on this concept—though his genetic approach did not allow him to arrive at its explicit formulation. But others who have continued and developed Freud's work—notably Franz Alexander, Otto Rank, Wilhelm Reich, and Harald Schultz-Hencke—have defined it more clearly. None of them, however, is agreed as to the precise nature and dynamics of this character structure.

My own starting point was a different one. Freud's postulations in regard to feminine psychology set me thinking about the role of cultural factors. Their influence on our ideas of what constitutes masculinity or femininity was obvious, and it became just as obvious to me that Freud had arrived at certain erroneous conclusions because he failed to take them into account. My interest in this subject grew over the course of fifteen years. It was furthered in part by association with Erich Fromm who, through his profound knowledge of both sociology and psychoanalysis, made me more aware of the significance of social factors over and above their circumscribed application to feminine psychology. And my impressions were confirmed when I came to the United States in 1932. I saw then that the attitudes and the neuroses of persons in this country differed in many ways from those I had observed in European countries, and that only the difference in civilizations could account for this. My conclusions finally found their expression in *The Neurotic Personality of Our Time.* The main contention here was that neuroses are brought about by cultural factors—which more specifically meant that neuroses are generated by disturbances in human relationships.

In the years before I wrote *The Neurotic Personality* I pursued another line of research that followed logically from the earlier hypothesis. It revolved around the question as to what the driving forces are in neurosis. Freud had been the first to point out that these were compulsive drives. He regarded these drives as instinctual in nature, aimed at satisfaction and intolerant of frustration. Consequently he believed that they were not confined to neuroses *per se* but operated in all human beings. If, however, neuroses were an outgrowth of disturbed human relationships, this postulation could not possibly be valid. The concepts I arrived at on this score were, briefly, these. Compulsive drives are specifically neurotic; they are born of feelings of isolation, helplessness, fear and hostility, and represent ways of coping with the world despite these feelings; they aim primarily not at satisfaction but at safety; their compulsive character is due to the anxiety lurking behind them. Two of these drives—neurotic cravings for affection and for power—stood out at first in clear relief and were presented in detail in *The Neurotic Personality*.

Though retaining what I considered the fundamentals of Freud's teachings, I realized by that time that my search for a better understanding had led me in directions that were at variance with Freud. If so many factors that Freud regarded as instinctual were culturally determined, if so much that Freud considered libidinal was a neurotic need for affection, provoked by anxiety and aimed at feeling safe with others, then the libido theory was no longer tenable. Childhood experiences remained important, but the influence they exerted on our lives appeared in a new light. Other theoretical differences inevitably followed. Hence it became necessary to formulate in my own mind where I stood in reference to Freud. The result of this clarification was *New Ways in Psychoanalysis*.

In the meantime my search for the driving forces in neurosis continued. I called the compulsive drives neurotic trends and described ten of them in my next book. By then I, too, had arrived at the point of recognizing that the neurotic character structure was of central significance. I regarded it at that time as a kind of macrocosm formed by many microcosms interacting upon one another. In the nucleus of each microcosm was a neurotic trend. This theory of neurosis had a practical application. If psychoanalysis did not primarily involve relating our present difficulties to our past experiences but depended rather upon understanding the interplay of forces in our existing personality, then recognizing and changing ourselves with little or even no expert help was entirely feasible. In the face of a widespread need for psychotherapy and a scarcity of available aid, self-analysis seemed to offer the hope of filling a vital need. Since the major part of the book dealt with the possibilities, limitations, and ways of analyzing ourselves, I called it *Self-Analysis.*

I was, however, not entirely satisfied with my presentation of individual trends. The trends themselves were accurately described; but I was haunted by the feeling that in a simple enumeration they appeared in a too isolated fashion. I could see that a neurotic need for affection, compulsive modesty, and the need for a "partner" belonged together. What I failed to see was that together they represented a basic attitude toward others and the self, and a particular philosophy of life. These trends are the nuclei of what I have now drawn together as a "moving toward people." I saw, too, that a compulsive craving for power and prestige and neurotic ambition had something in common. They constitute roughly the factors involved in what I shall call "moving against people." But the need for admiration and the perfectionist drives, though they had all the earmarks of neurotic trends and influenced the neurotic's relation with others, seemed primarily to concern his relations with himself. Also, the need for exploitation seemed to be less basic than either the need for affection or for power; it appeared less comprehensive than these, as if it were not a separate entity but had been taken out of some larger whole.

My questionings have since proved justified. In the years following, my focus of interest shifted to the role of conflicts in neurosis. I had said in *The Neurotic Personality* that a neurosis came about through the collision of divergent neurotic trends. In *Self-Analysis* I had said that neurotic trends not only reinforced each other but also created conflicts. Nevertheless conflicts had remained a side issue. Freud had been increasingly aware of the significance of inner conflicts; he saw them, however, as a battle between repressed and repressing forces. The conflicts I began to see were of a different kind. They operated between contradictory sets of neurotic trends, and though they originally concerned contradictory attitudes toward others, in time they encompassed contradictory attitudes toward the self, contradictory qualities and contradictory sets of values.

A crescendo of observation opened my eyes to the significance of such conflicts. What first struck me most forcibly was the blindness of patients toward obvious contradictions within themselves. When I pointed these out they became elusive and seemed to lose interest. After repeated experiences of this kind I realized that the elusiveness expressed a profound aversion to tackling these contradictions. Finally, panic reactions in response to a sudden recognition of a conflict showed me I was working with dynamite. Patients had good reason to shy away from these conflicts: they dreaded their power to tear them to pieces.

Then I began to recognize the amazing amount of energy and intelligence that was invested in more or less desperate efforts to "solve" [1] the conflicts or, more precisely, to deny their existence and create an artificial harmony. I saw the four major attempts at solution in about the order in which they are presented in this book. The initial attempt was to eclipse part of the conflict and raise its opposite to predominance. The second was to "move away from" people. The function of neurotic detachment now appeared in a new light. Detachment was part of the basic conflict—that is, one of the original conflicting attitudes toward others; but it also represented an attempt at solution, since maintaining an emotional distance between the self and others set the conflict out of operation. The third attempt was very different in kind. Instead of moving away from others, the neurotic moved away from himself. His whole actual self became somewhat unreal to him and he created in its place an idealized image of himself in which the conflicting parts were so transfigured that they no longer appeared as conflicts but as various aspects of a rich personality. This concept helped to clarify many neurotic problems which hitherto were beyond the reach of our understanding and hence of our therapy. It also put two of the neurotic trends which had previously resisted integration into their proper setting. The need for perfection now appeared as an endeavor to measure up to this idealized image; the craving for admiration could be seen as the patient's need to have outside affirmation that he really was his idealized image. And the farther the image was removed from reality the more insatiable this latter need would logically be. Of all the attempts at solution the idealized

[1] *See* footnote on page 33.

image is probably the most important by reason of its far-reaching effect on the whole personality. But in turn it generates a new inner rift, and hence calls for further patchwork. The fourth attempt at solution seeks primarily to do away with this rift, though it helps as well to spirit away all other conflicts. Through what I call externalization, inner processes are experienced as going on outside the self. If the idealized image means taking a step away from the actual self, externalization represents a still more radical divorce. It again creates new conflicts, or rather greatly augments the original conflict—that between the self and the outside world.

I have called these the four major attempts at solution, partly because they seem to operate regularly in all neuroses—though in varying degree—and partly because they bring about incisive changes in the personality. But they are by no means the only ones. Others of less general significance include such strategies as arbitrary rightness, whose main function is to quell all inner doubts; rigid self-control, which holds together a torn individual by sheer will power; and cynicism, which, in disparaging all values, eliminates conflicts in regard to ideals.

Meanwhile the consequences of all these unresolved conflicts were gradually becoming clearer to me. I saw the manifold fears that were generated, the waste of energy, the inevitable impairment of moral integrity, the deep hopelessness that resulted from feeling inextricably entangled.

It was only after I had grasped the significance of neurotic hopelessness that the meaning of sadistic trends finally came into view. These, I now understood, represented an attempt at restitution through vicarious living, entered upon by a person who despaired of ever being himself. And the all-consuming passion which can so often be observed in sadistic pursuits grew out of such a person's insatiable need for vindictive triumph. It became clear to me then that the need for destructive exploitation was in fact no separate neurotic trend but only a never-failing expression of that more comprehensive whole which for lack of a better term we call sadism.

Thus a theory of neurosis evolved, whose dynamic center is a basic conflict between the attitudes of "moving toward," "moving against," and "moving away from" people. Because of his fear of being split apart on the one hand and the necessity to function as a unity on the other, the neurotic makes desperate attempts at solution. While he can succeed this way in creating a kind of artificial equilibrium, new conflicts are constantly generated and further remedies are continually required to blot them out. Every step in this struggle for unity makes the neurotic more hostile, more helpless, more fearful, more alienated from himself and others, with the result that the difficulties responsible for the conflicts become more acute and their real resolution less and less attainable. He finally becomes hopeless and may try to find a kind of restitution in sadistic pursuits, which in turn have the effect of increasing his hopelessness and creating new conflicts.

This, then, is a fairly dismal picture of neurotic development and its resulting character structure. Why do I nonetheless call my theory a constructive one? In the first place it does away with the unrealistic optimism that maintains we can "cure" neuroses by absurdly simple means. But it involves no equally unrealistic pessimism. I call it constructive because it allows us for the first time to tackle and resolve neurotic hopelessness. I call it constructive most of all because in spite of its recognition of the severity of neurotic entanglements, it permits not only a tempering of the underlying conflicts but their actual resolution, and so enables us to work toward a real integration of personality. Neurotic conflicts cannot be resolved by rational decision. The neurotic's attempts at solution are not only futile but harmful. But these conflicts *can* be resolved by changing the conditions within the personality that brought them into being. Every piece of analytical work well done changes these conditions in that it makes a person less helpless, less fearful, less hostile, and less alienated from himself and others.

Freud's pessimism as regards neuroses and their treatment arose from the depths of his disbelief in human goodness and human growth. Man, he postulated, is doomed to suffer or to destroy. The instincts which drive him can only be controlled, or at best "sublimated." My own belief is that man has the capacity as well as the desire to develop his potentialities and become a decent human being, and that these deteriorate if his relationship to others and hence to himself is, and continues to be, disturbed. I believe that man can change and go on changing as long as he lives. And this belief has grown with deeper understanding.

PART I

*Neurotic Conflicts and
Attempts at Solution*

CHAPTER ONE

The Poignancy of Neurotic Conflicts

LET ME say to begin with: It is not neurotic to have conflicts. At one time or another our wishes, our interests, our convictions are bound to collide with those of others around us. And just as such clashes between ourselves and our environment are a commonplace, so, too, conflicts within ourselves are an integral part of human life.

An animal's actions are largely determined by instinct. Its mating, its care for its young, its search for food, its defenses against danger are more or less prescribed and beyond individual decision. In contrast, it is the prerogative as well as the burden of human beings to be able to exert choice, to have to make decisions. We may have to decide between desires that lead in opposite directions. We may, for instance, want to be alone but also want to be with a friend; we may want to study medicine but also to study music. Or there may be a conflict between wishes and obligations: we may wish to be with a lover when someone in trouble needs our care. We may be divided between a desire to be in accord with others and a conviction that would entail expressing an opinion antagonistic to them. We may be in conflict, finally, between two sets of values, as occurs when we believe in taking on a hazardous job in wartime but believe also in our duty to our family.

The kind, scope, and intensity of such conflicts are largely determined by the civilization in which we live. If the civilization is stable and tradition bound, the variety of choices presenting themselves are limited and the range of possible individual conflicts narrow. Even then they are not lacking. One loyalty may interfere with another; personal desires may stand against obligations to the group. But if the civilization is in a stage of rapid transition, where highly contradictory values and divergent ways of living exist side by side, the choices the individual has to make are manifold and difficult. He can conform to the expectations of the community or be a dissenting individualist, be gregarious or live as a recluse, worship success or despise it, have faith in strict discipline for children or allow them to grow up without much interference; he can believe in a different moral standard for men and women or hold that the same should apply for both, regard sexual relations as an expression of human intimacy or divorce them from ties of affection; he can foster racial discrimination or take the stand that human values are independent of the color of skin or the shape of noses—and so on and so forth.

There is no doubt that choices like these have to be made very often by people living in our civilization, and one would therefore expect conflicts along these lines to be quite common. But the striking fact is that most people are not aware of them, and consequently do not resolve them by any clear decision. More often than not they drift and let themselves be swayed by accident. They do not know where they stand; they make compromises without being aware of doing so; they are in-

volved in contradictions without knowing it. I am referring here to normal persons, meaning neither aver-
age nor ideal but merely non-neurotic.

There must, then, be preconditions for recognizing
contradictory issues and for making decisions on that
basis. These preconditions are fourfold. We must be
aware of what our wishes are, or even more, of what our
feelings are. Do we really like a person or do we only
think we like him because we are supposed to? Are we
really sad if a parent dies or do we only go through
the motions? Do we really wish to become a lawyer or
a doctor or does it merely strike us as a respectable and
profitable career? Do we really want our children to be
happy and independent or do we only give lip service
to the idea? Most of us would find it difficult to answer
such simple questions; that is, we do not know what we
really feel or want.

Since conflicts often have to do with convictions, beliefs, or moral values, their recognition would presup-
pose that we have developed our own set of values.
Beliefs that are merely taken over and are not a part
of us hardly have sufficient strength to lead to conflicts
or to serve as a guiding principle in making decisions.
When subjected to new influences, such beliefs will
easily be abandoned for others. If we simply have
adopted values cherished in our environment, conflicts
which in our best interest should arise do not arise.
If, for instance, a son has never questioned the wisdom
of a narrow-minded father, there will be little conflict
when the father wants him to enter a profession other
than the one he himself prefers. A married man who
falls in love with another woman is actually engaged in

a conflict; but when he has failed to establish his own convictions about the meaning of marriage he will simply drift along the path of least resistance instead of facing the conflict and making a decision one way or the other.

Even if we recognize a conflict as such, we must be willing and able to renounce one of the two contradictory issues. But the capacity for clear and conscious renunciation is rare, because our feelings and beliefs are muddled, and perhaps because in the last analysis most people are not secure and happy enough to renounce anything.

Finally, to make a decision presupposes the willingness and capacity to assume responsibility for it. This would include the risk of making a wrong decision and the willingness to bear the consequences without blaming others for them. It would involve feeling, "This is my choice, my doing," and presupposes more inner strength and independence than most people apparently have nowadays.

Caught as so many of us are in the strangling grip of conflicts—however unacknowledged—our inclination is to look with envy and admiration on people whose lives seem to flow along smoothly without being disturbed by any of this turbulence. The admiration may be warranted. These may be the strong ones who have established their own hierarchy of values, or who have acquired a measure of serenity because in the course of years conflicts and the need for decision have lost their uprooting power. But the outward appearance may be deceptive. More often, due to apathy, conformity, or opportunism, the people we envy are incapable of truly facing a conflict or of truly trying to resolve it on the basis of their own convictions, and consequently have merely drifted or been swayed by immediate advantage.

To experience conflicts knowingly, though it may be distressing, can be an invaluable asset. The more we face our own conflicts and seek out our own solutions, the more inner freedom and strength we will gain. Only when we are willing to bear the brunt can we approximate the ideal of being the captain of our ship. A spurious tranquillity rooted in inner dullness is anything but enviable. It is bound to make us weak and an easy prey to any kind of influence.

When conflicts center about the primary issues of life, it is all the more difficult to face them and resolve them. But provided we are sufficiently alive, there is no reason why in principle we should not be able to do so. Education could do much to help us to live with greater awareness of ourselves and to develop our own convictions. A realization of the significance of the factors involved in choice would give us ideals to strive for, and in that a direction for our lives.[1]

The difficulties always inherent in recognizing and resolving a conflict are immeasurably increased when a person is neurotic. Neurosis, it must be said, is always a matter of degree—and when I speak of "a neurotic" I invariably mean "a person to the extent that he is neurotic." For him awareness of feelings and desires is at a low ebb. Often the only feelings experienced con-

---

[1] To normal persons merely dulled by environmental pressures, a book like Harry Emerson Fosdick's *On Being a Real Person* would be of considerable profit.

sciously and clearly are reactions of fear and anger to blows dealt to vulnerable spots. And even these may be repressed. Such authentic ideals as do exist are so pervaded by compulsive standards that they are deprived of their power to give direction. Under the sway of these compulsive tendencies the faculty to renounce is rendered impotent, and the capacity to assume responsibility for oneself all but lost.[2]

Neurotic conflicts may be concerned with the same general problems as perplex the normal person. But they are so different in kind that the question has been raised whether it is permissible to use the same term for both. I believe it is, but we must be aware of the differences. What, then, are the characteristics of neurotic conflicts?

A somewhat simplified example by way of illustration: An engineer working in collaboration with others at mechanical research was frequently afflicted by spells of fatigue and irritability. One of these spells was brought about by the following incident. In a discussion of certain technical matters his opinions were less well received than those of his colleagues. Shortly afterward a decision was made in his absence, and no opportunity was given him subsequently to present his suggestions. Under these circumstances, he could have regarded the procedure as unjust and put up a fight, or he could have accepted the majority decision with good grace. Either reaction would have been consistent. But he did neither. Though he felt deeply slighted, he did not fight. Consciously he was merely aware of being irritated. The murderous rage within him appeared

[2] *Cf.* Chapter 10, Impoverishment of Personality.

only in his dreams. This repressed rage—a composite of his fury against the others and of his fury against himself for his own meekness—was mainly responsible for his fatigue.

His failure to react consistently was determined by a number of factors. He had built up a grandiose image of himself that required deference from others to support it. This was unconscious at the time: he simply acted on the premise that there was nobody as intelligent and competent in his field as he was. Any slight could jeopardize this premise and provoke rage. Furthermore, he had unconscious sadistic impulses to berate and humiliate others—an attitude so objectionable to him that he covered it up by overfriendliness. To this was added an unconsious drive to exploit people, making it imperative for him to keep in their good graces. The dependence on others was aggravated by a compulsive need for approval and affection, combined as it usually is with attitudes of compliance, appeasement, and avoidance of fight. There was thus a conflict between destructive aggressions—reactive rage and sadistic impulses—on the one hand, and on the other the need for affection and approval, with a desire to appear fair and rational in his own eyes. The result was inner upheaval that went unnoticed, while the fatigue that was its external manifestation paralyzed all action.

Looking at the factors involved in the conflict, we are struck first by their absolute incompatibility. It would be difficult indeed to imagine more extreme opposites than lordly demands for deference and ingratiating submissiveness. Second, the whole conflict remains unconscious. The contradictory tendencies operating in it are not recognized but are deeply repressed. Only slight bubbles of the battle raging within reach the surface. The emotional factors are rationalized: it is an injustice; it is a slight; my ideas were better. Third, the tendencies in both directions are compulsive. Even if he had some intellectual perception of his excessive demands, or of the existence and the nature of his dependence, he could not change these factors voluntarily. To be able to change them would require considerable analytical work. He was driven on either hand by compelling forces over which he had no control: he could not possibly renounce any of the needs acquired by stringent inner necessity. But none of them represented what he himself really wanted or sought. He would want neither to exploit nor to be submissive; as a matter of fact he despised these tendencies. Such a state of affairs, however, has a far-reaching significance for the understanding of neurotic conflicts. It means that no decision is feasible.

A further illustration presents a similar picture. A free-lance designer was stealing small sums of money from a good friend. The theft was not warranted by the external situation; he needed the money, but the friend would gladly have given it to him as he had on occasion in the past. That he should resort to stealing was particularly striking in that he was a decent fellow who set great store by friendship.

The following conflict was at the bottom of it. The man had a pronounced neurotic need for affection, especially a longing to be taken care of in all practical matters. Alloyed as this was with an unconscious drive to exploit others, his technique was to attempt both to endear and intimidate. These tendencies by themselves would have made him willing and eager to receive help and support. But he had also developed an extreme unconscious arrogance which involved a correspondingly vulnerable pride. Others should feel honored to be of service to him: it was humiliating for him to ask for help. His aversion to having to make a request was reinforced by a strong craving for independence and self-sufficiency that made it intolerable for him to admit he needed anything or to place himself under obligation. So he could take, but not receive.

The content of this conflict differs from that of the first example but the essential characteristics are the same. And any other example of neurotic conflict would show a like incompatibility of conflicting drives and their unconscious and compulsive nature, leading always to the impossibility of deciding between the contradictory issues involved.

Allowing for an indistinct line of demarcation, the difference, then, between normal and neurotic conflicts lies fundamentally in the fact that the disparity between the conflicting issues is much less great for the normal person than for the neurotic. The choices the former has to make are between two modes of action, either of which is feasible within the frame of a fairly integrated personality. Graphically speaking, the conflicting directions diverge only 90 degrees or less, as against the possible 180 degrees confronting the neurotic.

In awareness, too, the difference is one of degree. As

Kierkegaard [3] has pointed out: "Real life is far too multifarious to be portrayed by merely exhibiting such abstract contrasts as that between a despair which is completely unconscious, and one which is completely conscious." We can say this much, however: a normal conflict can be entirely conscious; a neurotic conflict in all its essential elements is always unconscious. Even though a normal person may be unaware of his conflict, he can recognize it with comparatively little help, while the essential tendencies producing a neurotic conflict are deeply repressed and can be unearthed only against great resistance.

The normal conflict is concerned with an actual choice between two possibilities, both of which the person finds really desirable, or between convictions, both of which he really values. It is therefore possible for him to arrive at a feasible decision even though it may be hard on him and require a renunciation of some kind. The neurotic person engulfed in a conflict is not free to choose. He is driven by equally compelling forces in opposite directions, neither of which he wants to follow. Hence a decision in the usual sense is impossible. He is stranded, with no way out. The conflict can only be resolved by working at the neurotic trends involved, and by so changing his relations with others and with himself that he can dispense with the trends altogether.

These characteristics account for the poignancy of neurotic conflicts. Not only are they difficult to recognize, not only do they render a person helpless, but they

[3] Søren Kierkegaard, *The Sickness unto Death*, Princeton University Press, 1941.

have as well a disruptive force of which he has good reason to be afraid. Unless we know these characteristics and keep them in mind, we shall not understand the desperate attempts at solution [4] which the neurotic enters upon, and which constitute the major part of a neurosis.

[4] Throughout the text I shall use the term "solve" in connection with the neurotic's attempts to do away with his conflicts. Since he unconsciously denies their existence he does not, strictly speaking, try to "resolve" them. His unconscious efforts are directed toward "solving" his problems.

CHAPTER TWO

The Basic Conflict

CONFLICTS play an infinitely greater role in neurosis than is commonly assumed. To detect them, however, is no easy matter—partly because they are essentially unconscious, but even more because the neurotic goes to any length to deny their existence. What, then, are the signals that would warrant us to suspect underlying conflicts? In the examples cited in the previous chapter their presence was indicated by two factors, both fairly obvious. One was the resulting symptoms—fatigue in the first case, stealing in the second. The fact is that every neurotic symptom points to an underlying conflict; that is, every symptom is a more or less direct outgrowth of a conflict. We shall see gradually what unresolved conflicts do to people, how they produce states of anxiety, depression, indecision, inertia, detachment, and so on. An understanding of the causative relation here helps direct our attention from the manifest disturbances to their source—though the exact nature of the source will not be disclosed.

The other signal indicating that conflicts were in operation was inconsistency. In the first example we saw a man convinced of a procedure being wrong and of injustice done him, making no move to protest. In the second a person who highly valued friendship turned to stealing money from a friend. Sometimes the person himself will be aware of such inconsistencies; more often he is blind to them even when they are blatantly obvious to an untrained observer.

Inconsistencies are as definite an indication of the presence of conflicts as a rise in body temperature is of physical disturbance. To cite some common ones: A girl wants above all else to marry, yet shrinks from the advances of any man. A mother oversolicitous of her children frequently forgets their birthdays. A person always generous to others is niggardly about small expenditures for himself. Another who longs for solitude never manages to be alone. One forgiving and tolerant toward most people is oversevere and demanding with himself.

Unlike the symptoms, the inconsistencies often permit of tentative assumptions as to the nature of the underlying conflict. An acute depression, for instance, reveals only the fact that a person is caught in a dilemma. But if an apparently devoted mother forgets her children's birthdays, we might be inclined to think that the mother was more devoted to her ideal of being a good mother than to the children themselves. We might also admit the possibility that her ideal collided with an unconscious sadistic tendency to frustrate them.

Sometimes a conflict will appear on the surface—that is, be consciously experienced as such. This would seem to contradict my assertion that neurotic conflicts are unconscious. But actually what appears is a distortion or modification of the real conflict. Thus a person may be torn by a conscious conflict when, in spite of his evasive techniques, well-functioning otherwise, he finds himself confronted with the necessity of making a major decision. He cannot decide now whether to marry this woman or that one or whether to marry at all, whether to take this or that job, whether to retain or dissolve a partnership. He will then go through the greatest torment, shuttling from one opposite to the other, utterly incapable of arriving at any decision. He may in his distress call upon an analyst, expecting him to clarify the particular issues involved. And he will necessarily be disappointed, because the present conflict is merely the point at which the dynamite of inner frictions finally exploded. The particular problem distressing him now cannot be solved without taking the long and tortuous road of recognizing the conflicts hidden beneath it.

In other instances the inner conflict may be externalized and appear in the person's conscious mind as an incompatibility between himself and his environment. Or, finding that seemingly unfounded fears and inhibitions interfere with his wishes, a person may be aware that the crosscurrents within himself issue from deeper sources.

The more knowledge we gain of a person, the better able we are to recognize the conflicting elements that account for the symptoms, inconsistencies, and surface conflicts—and, we must add, the more confusing becomes the picture, through the number and variety of contradictions. So we are led to ask: Can there be a basic conflict underlying all these particular conflicts and originally responsible for all of them? Can one picture the structure of conflict in terms, say, of an incompatible marriage, where an endless variety of apparently unrelated disagreements and rows over friends,

children, finances, mealtimes, servants, all point to some
fundamental disharmony in the relationship itself?

A belief in a basic conflict within the human personality is ancient and plays a prominent role in various
religions and philosophies. The powers of light and
darkness, of God and the devil, of good and evil are
some of the ways in which this belief has been expressed.
In modern psychology, Freud, on this score as on so
many others, has done pioneer work. His first assumption was that the basic conflict is one between our instinctual drives, with their blind urge for satisfaction,
and the forbidding environment—family and society.
The forbidding environment is internalized at an early
age and appears from then on as the forbidding superego.

It is hardly appropriate here to discuss this concept
with the seriousness it deserves. That would require
a recapitulation of all the arguments that have been
raised against the libido theory. Let us try rather to
understand the meaning of the concept itself, even if we
discard Freud's theoretical premises. What remains,
then, is the contention that the opposition between
primitive egocentric drives and our forbidding con-
science is the basic source of our manifold conflicts.
As will be seen later, I, too, attribute to this opposition
—or what is roughly comparable to it in my way of
thinking—a significant place in the structure of neuroses. What I dispute is its basic nature. My belief is
that though it is a major conflict, it is secondary and
arises of necessity during the development of a neurosis.

The reasons for this refutation will become apparent

later on. Just this one argument here: I do not believe that any conflict between desires and fears could ever account for the extent to which a neurotic is divided within himself and for an outcome so detrimental that it can actually ruin a person's life. A psychic situation such as Freud postulates would imply that a neurotic retains the capacity to strive for something wholeheart- edly, that he merely is frustrated in these strivings by the blocking action of fears. As I see it, the source of the conflict revolves around the neurotic's loss of capacity to wish for anything wholeheartedly because his very wishes are divided, that is, go in opposite directions.[1] This would constitute a much more serious condition indeed than the one Freud visualized.

In spite of the fact that I consider the fundamental conflict more disruptive than Freud does, my view of the possibility of an eventual solution is more positive than his. According to Freud, the basic conflict is uni- versal and in principle cannot be resolved: all that can be done is to arrive at better compromises or at better control. According to my view, the basic neurotic con- flict does not necessarily have to arise in the first place and is possible of resolution if it does arise—provided the sufferer is willing to undergo the considerable effort and hardship involved. This difference is not a matter of optimism or pessimism but inevitably results from the difference in our premises.

Freud's later answer to the question of a basic con- flict is philosophically quite appealing. Again setting

[1] *Cf.* Franz Alexander, "The Relation of Structural and In- stinctual Conflicts," *Psychoanalytic Quarterly,* Vol. XI, No. 2, April, 1933.

aside the various implications of his line of thought, his theory of a "life" and "death" instinct boils down to a conflict between constructive and destructive forces in human beings. Freud himself was less interested in bringing this concept to bear on conflicts than he was in the way the two forces are alloyed. He saw the possibility, for instance, of explaining masochistic and sadistic drives as a fusion between sexual and destructive instincts.

To apply this concept to the study of conflicts would have required the introduction of moral values. These, however, were to Freud illicit intruders in the realm of science. In line with his convictions, he strove to develop a psychology devoid of moral values. I believe that this very attempt to be "scientific" in the sense of the natural sciences is one of the more cogent reasons why Freud's theories and the therapy based on them are confined within too narrow channels. More specifically, it seems to have contributed to his failure to appreciate the role of conflicts in neurosis, despite his extensive work in this field.

Jung also placed considerable emphasis on the opposing tendencies in human beings. Indeed he was so impressed with the contradictions at work in the individual that he took it to be a general law that the presence of any element would of necessity indicate the presence also of its opposite. An outward femininity implied an inward masculinity; a surface extraversion, a concealed introversion; an outward preponderance of thinking and reasoning, an inner preponderance of feeling, and so on. Up to this point it would appear that Jung regarded conflicts as an essential feature of neurosis. However, he goes on to say that these opposites are not conflicting but complementary—the goal is to accept both and thereby approximate the ideal of wholeness. To him the neurotic is a person who has been stranded in a one-sided development. Jung formulated these concepts in what he called the law of complements. Now I, too, recognize that the opposing tendencies contain complementary elements neither of which can be dispensed with in an integrated personality. But in my opinion these are already outgrowths of neurotic conflicts and are so tenaciously adhered to because they represent attempts at solution. If, for instance, we regard a tendency toward being introspective, withdrawn, more concerned with one's own feelings, thoughts, or imagination than with other persons' as an authentic inclination—that is, constitutionally established and reinforced by experience—then Jung's reasoning would be correct. The effective therapeutic procedure would be to show the person his hidden "extravert" tendencies, to point out the dangers of one-sidedness in either direction, and encourage him to accept and live out both tendencies. If, however, we look upon introversion (or, as I prefer to call it, neurotic detachment) as a means of evading conflicts that arise in close contact with others, the task is not to encourage more extraversion but to analyze the underlying conflicts. The goal of wholeheartedness can be approximated only after these have been resolved.

Proceeding now to evolve my own position, I see the basic conflict of the neurotic in the fundamentally contradictory attitudes he has acquired toward other persons. Before going into detail, let me call attention to the dramatization of such a contradiction in the story of Dr. Jekyll and Mr. Hyde. We see him on the one hand delicate, sensitive, sympathetic, helpful, and on the other brutal, callous, and egotistical. I do not, of course, mean to imply that neurotic division always adheres to the precise line of this story, but merely to point to a vivid expression of basic incompatibility of attitudes in relation to others.

To approach the problem genetically we must go back to what I have called basic anxiety,[2] meaning by this the feeling a child has of being isolated and helpless in a potentially hostile world. A wide range of adverse factors in the environment can produce this insecurity in a child: direct or indirect domination, indifference, erratic behavior, lack of respect for the child's individual needs, lack of real guidance, disparaging attitudes, too much admiration or the absence of it, lack of reliable warmth, having to take sides in parental disagreements, too much or too little responsibility, overprotection, isolation from other children, injustice, discrimination, unkept promises, hostile atmosphere, and so on and so on.

The only factor to which I should like to draw special attention in this context is the child's sense of lurking hypocrisy in the environment: his feeling that the parents' love, their Christian charity, honesty, generosity, and so on may be only pretense. Part of what the child feels on this score is really hypocrisy; but some of it may be just his reaction to all the contradictions he

[2] Karen Horney, *The Neurotic Personality of Our Time,* W. W. Norton, 1937.

senses in the parents' behavior. Usually, however, there is a combination of cramping factors. They may be out in the open or quite hidden, so that in analysis one can only gradually recognize these influences on the child's development.

Harassed by these disturbing conditions, the child gropes for ways to keep going, ways to cope with this menacing world. Despite his own weakness and fears he unconsciously shapes his tactics to meet the particular forces operating in his environment. In doing so, he develops not only *ad hoc* strategies but lasting character trends which become part of his personality. I have called these "neurotic trends."

If we want to see how conflicts develop, we must not focus too sharply on the individual trends but rather take a panoramic view of the main directions in which a child can and does move under these circumstances. Though we lose sight for a while of details we shall gain a clearer perspective of the essential moves made to cope with the environment. At first a rather chaotic picture may present itself, but out of it in time three main lines crystallize: a child can move *toward* people, *against* them, or *away from* them.

When moving *toward* people he accepts his own helplessness, and in spite of his estrangement and fears tries to win the affection of others and to lean on them. Only in this way can he feel safe with them. If there are dissenting parties in the family, he will attach himself to the most powerful person or group. By complying with them, he gains a feeling of belonging and support which makes him feel less weak and less isolated.

When he moves *against* people he accepts and takes

for granted the hostility around him, and determines, consciously or unconsciously, to fight. He implicitly distrusts the feelings and intentions of others toward himself. He rebels in whatever ways are open to him. He wants to be the stronger and defeat them, partly for his own protection, partly for revenge.

against

When he moves *away from* people he wants neither to belong nor to fight, but keeps apart. He feels he has not much in common with them, they do not understand him anyhow. He builds up a world of his own—with nature, with his dolls, his books, his dreams.

away

In each of these three attitudes, one of the elements involved in basic anxiety is overemphasized: helplessness in the first, hostility in the second, and isolation in the third. But the fact is that the child cannot make any one of these moves wholeheartedly, because under the conditions in which the attitudes develop, all are bound to be present. What we have seen from our panoramic view is only the predominant move.

That this is so will become evident if we jump ahead now to the fully developed neurosis. We all know adults in whom one of the attitudes we have sketched stands out. But we can see, too, that his other tendencies have not ceased to operate. In a predominantly leaning and complying type we can observe aggressive propensities and some need for detachment. A predominantly hostile person has a compliant strain and needs detachment too. And a detached personality is not without hostility or a desire for affection.

The predominant attitude, however, is the one that most strongly determines actual conduct. It represents those ways and means of coping with others in which the particular person feels most at home. Thus a detached person will as a matter of course use all the unconscious techniques for keeping others at a safe distance because he feels at a loss in any situation that requires close association with them. Moreover, the ascendant attitude is often but not always the one most acceptable to the person's conscious mind.

This does not mean that the less conspicuous attitudes are less powerful. It would often be difficult to say, for instance, whether in an apparently dependent, compliant person the wish to dominate is of inferior intensity to the need for affection; his ways of expressing his aggressive impulses are merely more indirect. That the potency of the submerged tendencies may be very great is evidenced by the many instances in which the attitude accorded predominance is reversed. We can see such reversal in children, but it occurs in later life as well. Strickland in Somerset Maugham's *The Moon and Sixpence* would be a good illustration. Case histories of women often reveal this kind of change. A girl formerly tomboyish, ambitious, rebellious, when she falls in love may turn into a compliant, dependent woman, apparently without ambition. Or, under pressure of crushing experiences, a detached person may become morbidly dependent.

Changes like these, it should be added, throw some light on the frequent question whether later experience counts for nothing, whether we are definitely channeled, conditioned once and for all, by our childhood situation. Looking at neurotic development from the point of view of conflicts enables us to give a more adequate answer than is usually offered. These are the possibili-

ties: If the early situation is not too prohibitive of spontaneous growth, later experiences, particularly in adolescence, can have a molding influence. If, however, the
impact of early experiences has been powerful enough
to have molded the child to a rigid pattern, no new experience will be able to break through. In part this is
because his rigidity does not leave him open to any
new experience: his detachment, for instance, may be
too great to permit of anyone's coming close to him, or
his dependence so deep-rooted that he is forced always
to play a subordinate role and invite exploitation. In
part it is because he will interpret any new experience
in the language of his established pattern: the aggressive type, for instance, meeting with friendliness, will
view it either as a manifestation of stupidity or an attempt to exploit him; the new experience will tend
only to reinforce the old pattern. When a neurotic does
adopt a different attitude it may look as if later experiences had brought about a change in personality. However, the change is not as radical as it appears. Actually
what has happened is that combined internal and external pressures have forced him to abandon his predominant attitude in favor of the other extreme—but
this change would not have taken place if there had
been no conflicts to begin with.

From the point of view of the normal person there is
no reason why the three attitudes should be mutually
exclusive. One should be capable of giving in to others,
of fighting, and of keeping to oneself. The three can
complement each other and make for a harmonious

whole. If one predominates, it merely indicates an over-development along one line.

But in neurosis there are several reasons why these attitudes are irreconcilable. The neurotic is not flexible; he is driven to comply, to fight, to be aloof, regardless of whether the move is appropriate in the particular circumstance, and he is thrown into a panic if he behaves otherwise. Hence when all three attitudes are present in any strong degree, he is bound to be caught in a severe conflict.

Another factor, and one that considerably widens the scope of the conflict, is that the attitudes do not remain restricted to the area of human relationships but gradually pervade the entire personality, as a malignant tumor pervades the whole organic tissue. They end by encompassing not only the person's relation to others but also his relation to himself and to life in general. If we are not fully aware of this all-embracing character, the temptation is to think of the resulting conflict in categorical terms, like love *versus* hate, compliance *versus* defiance, submissiveness *versus* domination, and so on. That, however, would be as misleading as to distinguish fascism from democracy by focusing on any single opposing feature, such as their difference in approach to religion or power. These are differences certainly, but exclusive emphasis upon them would serve to obscure the point that democracy and fascism are worlds apart and represent two philosophies of life entirely incompatible with each other.

It is not accidental that a conflict that starts with our relation to others in time affects the whole personality. Human relationships are so crucial that they are bound to mold the qualities we develop, the goals we set for ourselves, the values we believe in. All these in turn react upon our relations with others and so are inextricably interwoven.[3]

My contention is that the conflict born of incompatible attitudes constitutes the core of neurosis and therefore deserves to be called *basic*. And let me add that I use the term *core* not merely in the figurative sense of its being significant but to emphasize the fact that it is the dynamic center from which neuroses emanate. This contention is the nucleus of a new theory of neurosis whose implications will become apparent in what follows. Broadly considered, the theory may be viewed as an elaboration of my earlier concept that neuroses are an expression of a disturbance in human relationships.[4]

[3] Since the relation to others and the attitude toward the self cannot be separated from one another, the contention occasionally to be found in psychiatric publications, that one or the other of these is the most important factor in theory and practice, is not tenable.

[4] This concept was first presented in *The Neurotic Personality of Our Time* and elaborated in *New Ways in Psychoanalysis* and *Self-Analysis.*

CHAPTER THREE

Moving Toward People

IT IS impossible to present the basic conflict by simply showing it in operation in a number of individuals. Because of its disruptive power the neurotic builds a defensive structure around it which serves not only to blot it from view but so deeply imbeds it that it cannot be isolated in pure form. The result is that what appears on the surface is more the various attempts at solution than the conflict itself. A simple detailing of case histories, therefore, would not bring all its implications and nuances into full relief; the presentation would necessarily be too circumstantial and give too untransparent a picture.

Besides, the outlines sketched in the preceding chapter need still to be filled in. To understand all that is involved in the basic conflict we must start by studying each of the opposing elements separately. We can do this with some success if we observe the types of individuals in whom one or the other element has become predominant, and for whom it represents the more acceptable self. For the sake of simplicity I shall classify such types as the compliant, the aggressive, and the detached personality.[1] We shall focus in each case on the

[1] The term "types" is used here merely as a simplification for persons with distinct characteristics. I definitely do not intend in this chapter or the two following to establish a new typology. A

person's more acceptable attitude, leaving out in so far
as possible the conflicts it conceals. In each of these
types we shall find that the basic attitude toward others
has created, or at least fostered, the growth of certain
needs, qualities, sensitivities, inhibitions, anxieties, and,
last but not least, a particular set of values.

This way of proceeding may have certain drawbacks,
but it also has definite advantages. By examining first
the functions and structure of a set of attitudes, reactions, beliefs, and so on in types where they are comparatively obvious, it will be easier to recognize similar
combinations in cases where they appear in somewhat
hazy and confused form. Furthermore, looking at the
undiluted picture will serve to bring into relief the
intrinsic incompatibility of the three attitudes. To come
back to our analogy of democracy *versus* fascism: If we
wanted to point out the essential difference between
democratic and fascist ideologies, we would not start by
presenting a person in whom a belief in certain democratic ideals was combined with a secret leaning toward
fascist methods. We would rather try first to get a picture of the fascist mind from National Socialist writings
and performance, and then proceed to compare these
with the most representative expressions of a democratic
way of life. This would give us a clear impression of the
contrast between the two sets of beliefs, and so help us
to understand persons and groups who have attempted
to effect a compromise between them.

Group I, the compliant type, manifests all the traits
that go with "moving toward" people. He shows a

typology is certainly desirable but must be established on a much
broader basis.

marked need for affection and approval and an especial
need for a "partner"—that is, a friend, lover, husband
or wife "who is to fulfill all expectations of life and take
responsibility for good and evil, his successful manipulation becoming the predominant task." [2] These needs
have the characteristics common to all neurotic trends;
that is, they are compulsive, indiscriminate, and generate anxiety or despondence when frustrated. They
operate almost independently of the intrinsic worth
of the "others" in question, as well as of the person's
real feeling toward them. However these needs may
vary in their expression, they all center around a desire
for human intimacy, a desire for "belonging." Because
of the indiscriminate nature of his needs, the compliant
type will be prone to overrate his congeniality and the
interests he has in common with those around him and
disregard the separating factors.[3] His misjudging of
people this way is not due to ignorance, stupidity, or
the inability to observe, but is determined by his compulsive needs. He feels—as illustrated by a patient's
drawing—like a baby surrounded by strange and threat-
ening animals. There she stood, tiny and helpless, in the
middle of the picture, around her a huge bee ready to
sting her, a dog that could bite her, a cat that could
jump at her, a bull that could gore her. Obviously, then,
the real nature of other beings does not matter, except
in so far as the more aggressive ones, being the more

[2] Quoted from Karen Horney, *Self-Analysis*, W. W. Norton,
1942.
[3] *Cf. The Neurotic Personality of Our Time, op. cit.*, Chapters
2 and 5, dealing with the need for affection, and *Self-Analysis,
op. cit.*, Chapter 8, dealing with morbid dependence.

frightening, are the ones whose "affection" is the most necessary. In sum, this type needs to be liked, wanted, desired, loved; to feel accepted, welcomed, approved of, appreciated; to be needed, to be of importance to others, especially to one particular person; to be helped, protected, taken care of, guided.

When in the course of analysis the compulsive character of these needs is pointed out to a patient, he will be likely to assert that all these desires are quite "natural." And, of course, here he is on defensible ground. Except for persons whose whole being has become so warped by sadistic trends (to be discussed later on) that the desire for affection is choked beyond all possibility of functioning, it is safe to assume that everyone does want to feel liked, to belong, to be helped, and so on. Where the patient errs is in claiming that all his frantic beating about for affection and approval is genuine, while in reality the genuine portion is heavily overshadowed by his insatiable urge to feel safe.

The need to satisfy this urge is so compelling that everything he does is oriented toward its fulfillment. In the process he develops certain qualities and attitudes that mold his character. Some of these could be called endearing: he becomes sensitive to the needs of others —within the frame of what he is able to understand emotionally. For example, though he is likely to be quite oblivious to a detached person's wish to be aloof, he will be alert to another's need for sympathy, help, approval, and so on. He tries automatically to live up to the expectations of others, or to what he believes to be their expectations, often to the extent of losing sight of his own feelings. He becomes "unselfish," self-sacri-

ficing, undemanding—except for his unbounded desire
for affection. He becomes compliant, overconsiderate—
within the limits possible for him—overappreciative,
overgrateful, generous. He blinds himself to the fact
that in his heart of hearts he does not care much for
others and tends to regard them as hypocritical and self-
seeking. But—if I may use conscious terms for what goes
on unconsciously—he persuades himself that he likes
everyone, that they are all "nice" and trustworthy, a
fallacy which not only makes for heartbreaking disappointments but adds to his general insecurity.

These qualities are not as valuable as they appear to
the person himself, particularly since he does not con-
sult his own feelings or judgment but gives blindly to
others all that he is driven to want from them—and
because he is profoundly disturbed if the returns fail
to materialize.

Along with these attributes and overlapping them
goes another lot, aimed at avoiding black looks, quarrels, competition. He tends to subordinate himself,
takes second place, leaving the limelight to others; he
will be appeasing, conciliatory, and—at least consciously
—bears no grudge. Any wish for vengeance or triumph
is so profoundly repressed that he himself often wonders at his being so easily reconciled and at his never
harboring resentment for long. Important in this context is his tendency automatically to shoulder blame.
Again quite regardless of his real feelings—that is,
whether he really feels guilty or not—he will accuse
himself rather than others and tend to scrutinize himself or be apologetic in the face of obviously unwarranted criticism or anticipated attack.

There is an imperceptible transition from these attitudes to definite inhibitions. Because any kind of aggressive behavior is taboo, we find here inhibitions in regard to being assertive, critical, demanding, giving orders, making an impression, striving for ambitious goals. Also, because his life is altogether oriented toward others, his inhibitions often prevent him from doing things for himself or enjoying things by himself. This may reach a point where any experience not shared with someone—whether a meal, a show, music, nature—becomes meaningless. Needless to say, such a rigid restriction on enjoyment not only impoverishes life but makes dependence on others all the greater.

Apart from his idealization [4] of the qualities just named, this type has certain characteristic attitudes toward himself. One is the pervasive feeling that he is weak and helpless—a "poor little me" feeling. When left to his own resources he feels lost, like a boat loosed from its moorings, or like Cinderella bereft of her fairy godmother. This helplessness is in part real; certainly the feeling that under no circumstances could one possibly fight or compete does promote actual weakness. Besides, he frankly admits his helplessness to himself and others. It may be dramatically emphasized in dreams as well. He often resorts to it as a means of appeal or defense: "You must love me, protect me, forgive me, not desert me, *because* I am so weak and helpless."

A second characteristic grows out of his tendency to subordinate himself. He takes it for granted that everyone is superior to him, that they are more attractive, more intelligent, better educated, more worth while

[4] *Cf.* Chapter 6, The Idealized Image.

than he. There is factual basis for this feeling in that his lack of assertiveness and firmness does impair his capacities; but even in fields where he is unquestionably able his feeling of inferiority leads him to credit the other fellow—regardless of his merit—with greater competence than his own. In the presence of aggressive or arrogant persons his sense of his own worthiness shrinks still more. However, even when alone his tendency is to undervalue not only his qualities, talents, and abilities but his material possessions as well.

A third typical feature is a part of his general dependence upon others. This is his unconscious tendency to rate himself by what others think of him. His self-esteem rises and falls with their approval or disapproval, their affection or lack of it. Hence any rejection is actually catastrophic for him. If someone fails to return an invitation he may be reasonable about it consciously, but in accordance with the logic of the particular inner world in which he lives, the barometer of his self-esteem drops to zero. In other words any criticism, rejection, or desertion is a terrifying danger, and he may make the most abject effort to win back the regard of the person who has thus threatened him. His offering of the other cheek is not occasioned by some mysterious "masochistic" drive but is the only logical thing he can do on the basis of his inner premises.

All of this contributes to his special set of values. Naturally, the values themselves are more or less lucid and confirmed according to his general maturity. They lie in the direction of goodness, sympathy, love, generosity, unselfishness, humility; while egotism, ambition, callousness, unscrupulousness, wielding of power are abhorred—though these attributes may at the same time be secretly admired because they represent "strength."

These, then, are the elements involved in a neurotic "moving toward" people. It must be apparent now how inadequate it would be to describe them by any *one* term like submissive or dependent, for a whole way of thinking, feeling, acting—a whole way of life—is implicit in them.

I promised not to discuss the contradictory factors. But we will not fully understand how rigidly all the attitudes and beliefs are adhered to unless we are aware of the extent to which the repression of opposing trends reinforces the dominant ones. So we shall take a brief glance at the reverse side of the picture. When analyzing the compliant type we find a variety of aggressive tendencies strongly repressed. In decided contrast to the apparent oversolicitude, we come upon a callous lack of interest in others, attitudes of defiance, unconscious parasitic or exploiting tendencies, propensities to control and manipulate others, relentless needs to excel or to enjoy vindictive triumphs. Naturally the repressed drives vary in kind and intensity. In part they arise in response to early unfortunate experiences with others. A history will, for instance, frequently show temper tantrums up to the age of five or eight, disappearing then to give place to a general docility. But aggressive trends are also reinforced and fed by later experience, since hostility is continually generated from many sources. It would lead us too far afield to go into all of these at this point; suffice it to say here that self-effacement and "goodness" invite being stepped on and being taken advantage of; further, that dependence upon others makes for exceptional vulnerability, which in turn leads to a feeling of being neglected, rejected, and humiliated whenever the excessive amount of affection or approval demanded is not forthcoming.

When I say that all these feelings, drives, attitudes are "repressed" I use the term in Freud's sense, meaning that the individual is not only unaware of them but has so implacable an interest in never becoming aware of them that he keeps anxious watch lest any traces be disclosed to himself or others. Every repression thus confronts us with the question: What interest has the individual in repressing certain forces operating within him? In the case of the compliant type we can find several answers. Most of them we can understand only later when we come to discuss the idealized image and sadistic trends. What we can already understand at this point is that feelings or expressions of hostility would endanger the person's need to like others and to be liked by them. In addition, any kind of aggressive or even self-assertive behavior would appear to him as selfish. He would condemn it himself and hence would feel that others condemned it, too. And he cannot afford to risk such condemnation because his self-esteem is all too dependent upon their approval.

The repression of all assertive, vindictive, ambitious feelings and impulses has still another function. It is one of the many attempts a neurotic makes to do away with his conflicts and to create instead a feeling of unity, of oneness, of wholeness. The longing for unity within ourselves is no mystical desire but is prompted by the practical necessity of having to function in life—an impossibility when one is continually driven in opposite directions—and by what in consequence amounts to a supreme terror of being split apart. Giving predominance to one trend by submerging all discrepant elements is an unconscious attempt to organize the personality. It constitutes one of the major attempts to solve neurotic conflicts.

So we have already discovered a twofold interest in keeping a strict check on all aggressive impulses: the person's whole way of life would be endangered and his artificial unity exploded. And the more destructive the aggressive trends, the more stringent the necessity to exclude them. The individual will lean over backward never to appear to want anything for himself, never to refuse a request, always to like everyone, always to keep in the background, and so on. In other words, the compliant, appeasing trends are reinforced; they become more compulsive and less discriminate.[5]

Naturally, all these unconscious efforts do not keep the repressed impulses from operating or asserting themselves. But they do so in ways that fit into the structure. The person will make demands "because he is so miserable" or will secretly dominate under the guise of "loving." Accumulated repressed hostility may also appear in explosions of greater or less vehemence, ranging from occasional irritability to temper tantrums. These outbursts, while they do not fit into the picture of gentleness and mildness, appear to the individual himself as entirely justified. And according to his premises he is quite right. Not knowing that his demands upon others are excessive and egocentric, he cannot help feeling at times that he is so unfairly treated that he simply can't

[5] *Cf.* Chapter 12, Sadistic Trends.

stand it any longer. Finally, if the repressed hostility takes on the force of a blind fury, it may give rise to all kinds of functional disorders, like headaches or stomach ailments.

Most of the characteristics of the compliant type thus have a double motivation. When he subordinates himself, for instance, it is in the interest of avoiding friction and thereby achieving harmony with others; but it may also be a means of eradicating all traces of his need to excel. When he lets others take advantage of him it is an expression of compliance and "goodness," but it may also be a turning away from his own wish to exploit. For neurotic compliance to be overcome, both sides of the conflict must be worked through, and in the proper order. From conservative psychoanalytic publications we sometimes get the impression that the "liberation of aggressions" is the essence of psychoanalytic therapy. Such an approach shows little understanding of the complexities and particularly of the variations in neurotic structures. Only for the particular type under discussion does it have any validity, and even here the validity is limited. The uncovering of aggressive drives is liberating, but it can easily be detrimental to the person's development if the "liberation" is regarded as an end in itself. It must be followed by a working through of the conflicts, if the personality is ultimately to be integrated.

We need still to turn our attention to the role that love and sex play for the compliant type. Love often appears to him as the only goal worth striving for, worth living for. Life without love appears flat, futile, empty. To use a phrase Fritz Wittels has applied to compulsive pursuits,[6] love becomes a phantom that is chased to the exclusion of everything else. People, nature, work, or any kind of amusement or interest become utterly meaningless unless there is some love relationship to lend them flavor and zest. The fact that under the conditions of our civilization this obsession is more frequent and more apparent in women than in men has given rise to the notion that it is a specifically feminine longing. Actually, it has nothing to do with femininity or masculinity but is a neurotic phenomenon in that it is an irrational compulsive drive.

If we understand the structure of the compliant type we can see why love is so all important to him, why there is "method in his madness." In view of his contradictory compulsive tendencies, it is in fact the only way in which all his neurotic needs can be fulfilled. It promises to satisfy the need to be liked as well as to dominate (through love), the need to take second place as well as to excel (through the partner's undivided regard). It permits him to live out all his aggressive drives on a justified, innocent, or even praiseworthy basis, while allowing him at the same time to express all the endearing qualities he has acquired. Furthermore, since he is unaware that his handicaps and his suffering issue from the conflicts within himself, love beckons as the sure cure for them all: if only he can find a person who loves him, *everything* will be all right. It is easy enough to say that this hope is fallacious, but we must also understand the logic of his more or less unconscious reasoning. He thinks: "I am weak and helpless; as long

[6] Fritz Wittels, "Unconscious Phantoms in Neurotics," *Psychoanalytic Quarterly,* Vol. VIII, Part 2, 1939.

as I am alone in this hostile world, my helplessness is a danger and a threat. But if I find someone who loves me above all others, I shall no longer be in danger, for he (she) will protect me. With him I shouldn't need to assert myself, for he would understand and give me what I want without my having to ask or explain. In fact, my weakness would be an asset, because he would love my helplessness and I could lean on his strength. The initiative which I simply can't muster for myself would flourish if it meant doing things for him, or even doing things for myself because he wanted it."

He thinks—again reconstructing in terms of formulated reasoning what is partly thought out, partly only a feeling, and partly quite unconscious: "It is torture for me to be alone. It's not only that I can't enjoy anything I do not share. It's more than that; I feel lost, I feel anxious. Surely I could go to a movie alone or read a book on a Saturday night, but that would be humiliating because it would point out to me that nobody wants me. So I must plan carefully never to be alone on a Saturday evening—or at any other time, for that matter. But if I found the great lover, he would free me from this torture; I would never be alone; everything that is now meaningless, whether it's preparing breakfast or working or seeing a sunset, would be a joy."

And he thinks: "I have no self-confidence. I always feel everybody else is more competent, more attractive, more gifted than I am. Even the things I've managed to accomplish don't count, because I can't really credit myself with them. I may have been bluffing, or it may have been just a lucky break. I certainly can't be sure that I could do it again. And if people really knew me,

they'd have no use for me anyway. But if I found someone who loved me as I am and to whom I was of prime
importance, I would be somebody." No wonder, then,
that love has all the lure of a mirage. No wonder that it
should be clutched at in preference to the laborious
process of changing from within.

Sexual intercourse as such—aside from its biological
function—has the value of constituting proof of being
wanted. The more the compliant type tends to be detached—that is, afraid of being emotionally involved—or
the more he despairs of being loved, the more will mere
sexuality be likely to substitute for love. It will then
appear as the only road to human intimacy, and be over-
rated, as love is, for its power to solve everything.

If we are careful to avoid both extremes—that of regarding the patient's overemphasis on love as "only
natural," and that of dismissing it as "neurotic"—we
shall see that the compliant type's expectations in this
direction come as a logical conclusion from his philosophy of life. As so often in neurotic phenomena—or is
it always?—we find that the patient's reasoning, conscious or unconscious, is flawless, but rests on false
premises. The fallacious premises are that he mistakes
his need for affection and all that goes with it for a
genuine capacity to love, and that he completely leaves
out of the equation his aggressive and even destructive
trends. In other words he leaves out the whole neurotic
conflict. What he expects is to do away with the harmful consequences of the unresolved conflicts without
changing anything in the conflicts themselves—an attitude characteristic of every neurotic attempt at solution.
That is why these attempts are inevitably doomed to

failure. For love as a solution, one must say this, however. If the compliant type is fortunate enough to find a partner who has both strength and kindliness, or whose neurosis fits in with his own, his suffering may be considerably lessened and he may find a moderate amount of happiness. But as a rule, the relationship from which he expects heaven on earth only plunges him into deeper misery. He is all too likely to carry his conflicts into the relationship and thereby destroy it. Even the most favorable possibility can relieve only the actual distress; unless his conflicts are resolved his development will still be blocked.

CHAPTER FOUR

Moving Against People

IN DISCUSSING the second aspect of the basic conflict—the tendency to "move against" people—we shall proceed as before, examining here the type in whom aggressive trends predominate.

Just as the compliant type clings to the belief that people are "nice," and is continually baffled by evidence to the contrary, so the aggressive type takes it for granted that everyone is hostile, and refuses to admit that they are not. To him life is a struggle of all against all, and the devil take the hindmost. Such exceptions as he allows are made reluctantly and with reservation. His attitude is sometimes quite apparent, but more often it is covered over with a veneer of suave politeness, fair-mindedness and good fellowship. This "front" can represent a Machiavellian concession to expediency. As a rule, however, it is a composite of pretenses, genuine feelings, and neurotic needs. A desire to make others believe he is a good fellow may be combined with a certain amount of actual benevolence as long as there is no question in anybody's mind that he himself is in command. There may be elements of a neurotic need for affection and approval, put to the service of aggressive goals. No such "front" is necessary to the compliant type because his values coincide anyway with approved-of social or Christian virtues.

To appreciate the fact that the needs of the aggressive type are just as compulsive as those of the compliant, we must realize that they are as much prompted by basic anxiety as his. This must be emphasized, because the component of fear, so evident in the latter, is never admitted or displayed by the type we are now considering. In him everything is geared toward being, becoming, or at least appearing tough.

His needs stem fundamentally from his feeling that the world is an arena where, in the Darwinian sense, only the fittest survive and the strong annihilate the weak. What contributes most to survival depends largely on the civilization in which the person lives; but in any case, a callous pursuit of self-interest is the paramount law. Hence his primary need becomes one of control over others. Variations in the means of control are infinite. There may be an outright exercise of power, there may be indirect manipulation through oversolicitousness or putting people under obligation. He may prefer to be the power behind the throne. The approach may be by way of the intellect, implying a belief that by reasoning or foresight everything can be managed. His particular form of control depends partly on his natural endowments. Partly, it represents a fusion of conflicting trends. If, for instance, the person inclines at the same time toward detachment he will shun any direct domination because it brings him into too close contact with others. Indirect methods will also be preferred if there is much hidden need for affection. If his wish is to be the power behind the throne, the presence of sadistic trends is indicated, since it implies using others for the attainment of one's goals.[1]

[1] *Cf.* Chapter 12, Sadistic Trends.

Concomitantly he needs to excel, to achieve success, prestige, or recognition in any form. Strivings in this direction are partly oriented toward power, inasmuch as success and prestige lend power in a competitive society. But they also make for a subjective feeling of strength through outside affirmation, outside acclaim, and the fact of supremacy. Here as in the compliant type the center of gravity lies outside the person himself; only the kind of affirmation wanted from others differs. Factually the one is as futile as the other. When people wonder why success has failed to make them feel any less insecure, they only show their psychological ignorance, but the fact that they do so indicates the extent to which success and prestige are commonly regarded as yardsticks.

A strong need to exploit others, to outsmart them, to make them of use to himself, is part of the picture. Any situation or relationship is looked at from the standpoint of "What can I get out of it?"—whether it has to do with money, prestige, contacts, or ideas. The person himself is consciously or semiconsciously convinced that everyone acts this way, and so what counts is to do it more efficiently than the rest. The qualities he develops are almost diametrically opposed to those of the compliant type. He becomes hard and tough, or gives that appearance. He regards all feelings, his own as well as others', as "sloppy sentimentality." Love, for him, plays a negligible role. Not that he is never "in love" or never has an affair or marries, but what is of prime concern is to have a mate who is eminently desirable, one through whose attractiveness, social prestige, or wealth he can enhance his own position. He sees no reason to be considerate of others. "Why should I care

—let others take care of themselves." In terms of the old ethical problem of two persons on a raft only one of whom could survive, he would say that of course he'd try to save his own skin—not to would be stupid and hypocritical. He hates to admit fear of any kind and will find drastic ways of bringing it under control. He might, for instance, force himself to stay in an empty house although he is terrified of burglars; he might insist on riding horseback until he has overcome his fear of horses; he might intentionally walk through swamps where there are known to be snakes in order to rid himself of his terror of them.

While the compliant type tends to appease, the aggressive type does everything he can to be a good fighter. He is alert and keen in an argument and will go out of his way to launch one for the sake of proving he is right. He may be at his best when his back is to the wall and there is no alternative but to fight. In contrast to the compliant type who is afraid to win a game, he is a bad loser and undeniably wants victory. He is just as ready to accuse others as the former is to take blame on himself. In neither case does the consideration of guilt play a role. The compliant type when he pleads guilty is by no means convinced that he is so, but is driven to appease. The aggressive type similarly is not convinced that the other fellow is wrong; he just assumes he is right because he needs this ground of subjective certainty in much the same way as an army needs a safe point from which to launch an attack. To admit an error when it is not absolutely necessary seems to him an unforgivable display of weakness, if not arrant fool- ishness.

It is consistent with his attitude of having to fight against a malevolent world that he should develop a keen sense of realism—of its kind. He will never be so "naïve" as to overlook in others any manifestation of ambition, greed, ignorance, or anything else that might obstruct his own goals. Since in a competitive civilization attributes like these are much more common than real decency, he feels justified in regarding himself as only realistic. Actually, of course, he is just as one-sided as the compliant type. Another facet of his realism is his emphasis on planning and foresight. Like any good strategist, in every situation he is careful to appraise his own chances, the forces of his adversaries, and the possible pitfalls.

Because he is driven always to assert himself as the strongest, shrewdest, or most sought after, he tries to develop the efficiency and resourcefulness necessary to being so. The zest and intelligence he puts into his work may make him a highly esteemed employee or a success in a business of his own. However, the impression he gives of having an absorbing interest in his work will in a sense be misleading, because for him work is only a means to an end. He has no love for what he is doing and takes no real pleasure in it—a fact consistent with his attempt to exclude feelings from his life altogether. This choking off of all feeling has a two-edged effect. On the one hand it is undoubtedly expedient from the standpoint of success in that it enables him to function like a well-oiled machine, untiringly producing the goods that will bring him ever more power and prestige. Here feelings might interfere. They could conceivably lead him into a line of work with fewer opportunistic advantages; they might cause him to shy away from the techniques so often employed on the road to success; they might tempt him away from his work to the enjoyment of nature or art, or to the companionship of friends instead of persons merely useful to his purpose. On the other hand the emotional barrenness that results from a throttling of feeling will do something to the quality of his work; certainly it is bound to detract from his creativity.

The aggressive type looks like an exquisitely uninhibited person. He can assert his wishes, he can give orders, express anger, defend himself. But actually he has no fewer inhibitions than the compliant type. It is not greatly to the credit of our civilization that his particular inhibitions do not, offhand, strike us as such. They lie in the emotional area and concern his capacity for friendship, love, affection, sympathetic understanding, disinterested enjoyment. The last he would set down as a waste of time.

His feeling about himself is that he is strong, honest, and realistic, all of which is true if you look at things his way. According to his premises his estimate of himself is strictly logical, since to him ruthlessness is strength, lack of consideration for others, honesty, and a callous pursuit of one's own ends, realism. His attitude on the score of his honesty comes partly from a shrewd debunking of current hypocrisies. Enthusiasm for a cause, philanthropic sentiments, and the like he sees as sheer pretense, and it is not hard for him to expose gestures of social consciousness or Christian virtue for what they so often are. His set of values is built around the philosophy of the jungle. Might makes right. Away with humaneness and mercy. *Homo homini lupus.* Here we have values not very different from those with which the nazis have made us so familiar.

There is subjective logic in the tendency of the aggressive type to reject real sympathy and friendliness as well as their counterfeits, compliance and appeasement. But it would be a mistake to assume that he cannot tell the difference. When he meets with an indubitably friendly spirit coupled with strength he is well able to recognize and respect it. The point is that he believes it to be against his interest to be too discriminating in this respect. Both attitudes strike him as liabilities in the battle for survival.

Why, though, does he reject the softer human sentiments with such violence? Why is he likely to feel nauseated at the sight of affectionate behavior in others? Why is he so contemptuous when someone shows sympathy at what he considers the wrong moment? He acts like the man who chased beggars from his door because they were breaking his heart. He may indeed literally be abusive to beggars; he may refuse the simplest request with a vehemence quite out of proportion. Reactions like these are typical of him and can readily be observed as the aggressive trends become less rigid during analysis. Actually, his feelings on the score of "softness" in others are mixed. He despises it in them, it is true, but he welcomes it as well, because it leaves him all the freer to pursue his own goals. Why else should he so often feel drawn toward the compliant type—just as the latter is so often drawn toward him? The reason his reaction is so extreme is that it is prompted by his need to fight all softer feelings within himself. Nietzsche gives us a good illustration of these dynamics when he has his superman see any form of sympathy as a sort of fifth column, an enemy operating from within. "Softness" to this kind of person means not only genuine affection, pity, and the like but everything implicit in the needs, feelings, and standards of the compliant type. In the case of the beggar, for instance, he would have stirrings of real sympathy, a need to comply with the request, a feeling that he ought to be helpful. But there is a still greater need to push all this away from him, with the result that he not only refuses but abuses.

The hope of fusing his divergent drives, which the compliant type places in love, is sought by the aggressive in recognition. To be recognized promises him not only the affirmation of himself he requires but holds out the additional lure of being liked by others and of being able in turn to like them. Since recognition thus appears to offer solution of his conflicts, it becomes the saving mirage he pursues.

The inner logic of his struggle is in principle identical with that presented in the case of the compliant type and therefore need only be briefly indicated here. For the aggressive type any feeling of sympathy, or obligation to be "good," or attitude of compliance would be incompatible with the whole structure of living he has built up and would shake its foundations. Moreover, the emergence of these opposing tendencies would confront him with his basic conflict and so destroy the organization he has carefully nurtured—the organization for unity. The consequence will be that repression of the softer tendencies will reinforce the aggressive ones, making them all the more compulsive.

If the two types we have discussed are now vivid in our minds we can see that they represent polar extremes. What is desirable to one is abhorrent to the other. The one has to like everyone, the other to regard all as potential enemies. The one seeks to avoid fight at all costs, the other finds it is his natural element. The one clings to fear and helplessness, the other tries to dismiss them. The one moves, however neurotically, toward humane ideals, the other toward the philosophy of the jungle. But all the while neither of these patterns is freely chosen: each is compulsive and inflexible, determined by inner necessities. There is no middle ground on which they can meet.

We are ready now to take the step our presentation of types has led up to, and for the sake of which we have discussed them. We set out to discover just what the basic conflict involved, and so far have seen two aspects of it operating as predominant trends in two distinct types. The step we must now take is to picture a person in whom these two opposite sets of attitudes and values are equally at work. Is it not clear that such a person would be so inexorably driven in two diametrically opposite directions that he would hardly be able to function at all? The fact of the matter is that he would be split and paralyzed beyond all power to act. It is his effort to eliminate one set that puts him into one or the other of the categories we have described; it is one of the ways he attempts to solve his conflicts.

To speak as Jung does, in such a case, of a one-sided

development appears thoroughly inadequate. It is at best a formalistically correct statement. But since it is based on a misconception of the dynamics, the implications are wrong. When Jung, starting from the concept of one-sidedness, continues to say that in therapy the patient must be helped to accept his opposite side, we say: How is that possible? The patient cannot accept it, he can only recognize it. If Jung expects this step to make him a whole person, we should reply that certainly this step is necessary to eventual integration, but of itself it merely means a facing of his conflicts, which hitherto he has avoided. What Jung has not properly evaluated is the compulsive nature of neurotic trends. Between moving toward people and moving against people there is not simply the difference between weakness and strength—or, as Jung would say, between femininity and masculinity. We all have potentialities both for compliance and aggression. And if a person not compulsively driven struggles hard enough, he can arrive at some integration. When the two patterns are neurotic, however, both are harmful to our growth. Two undesirables added together do not make a desirable whole, nor can two incompatibles make a harmonious entity.

CHAPTER FIVE

Moving Away From People

THE THIRD face of the basic conflict is the need for detachment, for "moving away from" people. Before examining it in the type for whom it has become the predominant trend, we must understand what is meant by neurotic detachment. Certainly it is not the mere fact of wanting occasional solitude. Everyone who takes himself and life seriously wants to be alone at times. Our civilization has so engulfed us in the externals of living that we have little understanding of this need, but its possibilities for personal fulfillment have been stressed by philosophies and religions of all times. A desire for meaningful solitude is by no means neurotic; on the contrary most neurotics shrink from their own inner depths, and an incapacity for constructive solitude is itself a sign of neurosis. Only if there is intolerable strain in associating with people and solitude becomes primarily a means of avoiding it is the wish to be alone an indication of neurotic detachment.

Certain of the highly detached person's peculiarities are so characteristic of him that psychiatrists are inclined to think of them as belonging exclusively to the detached type. The most obvious of these is a general estrangement from people. In him this strikes our attention because he particularly emphasizes it, but actually his estrangement is no greater than that of other neurotics. In the case of the two types we have discussed, for instance, it would be impossible to make a general statement as to which was the more estranged. We can only say that this characteristic is covered over in the compliant type, that he is surprised and frightened when he discovers it, because his passionate need for closeness makes him so eager to believe that no gap between himself and others exists. After all, estrangement from people is only an indication that human relationships are disturbed. But this is the case in all neuroses. The extent of the estrangement depends more on the severity of the disturbance than on the particular form the neurosis takes.

Another characteristic that is often regarded as peculiar to detachment is estrangement from the self, that is, a numbness to emotional experience, an uncertainty as to what one is, what one loves, hates, desires, hopes, fears, resents, believes. Such self-estrangement is again common to all neuroses. Every person, to the extent that he is neurotic, is like an airplane directed by remote control and so bound to lose touch with himself. Detached persons can be quite like the zombies of Haitian lore—dead, but revived by witchcraft: they can work and function like live persons, but there is no life in them. Others, again, can have a comparatively rich emotional life. Since such variations exist, we cannot regard self-estrangement, either, as exclusive to detachment. What all detached persons have in common is something quite different. It is their capacity to look at themselves with a kind of objective interest, as one would look at a work of art. Perhaps the best way to describe it would be to say that they have the same "on-

looker" attitude toward themselves that they have toward life in general. They may often, therefore, be
excellent observers of the processes going on within
them. An outstanding example of this is the uncanny
understanding of dream symbols they frequently display.

What is crucial is their inner need to put emotional
distance between themselves and others. More accurately, it is their conscious and unconscious determination not to get emotionally involved with others in any
way, whether in love, fight, co-operation, or competition. They draw around themselves a kind of magic
circle which no one may penetrate. And this is why,
superficially, they may "get along" with people. The
compulsive character of the need shows up in their reaction of anxiety when the world intrudes on them.

All the needs and qualities they acquire are directed
toward this major need of not getting involved. Among
the most striking is a need for *self-sufficiency*. Its most
positive expression is resourcefulness. The aggressive
type also tends to be resourceful—but the spirit is different; for him it is a prerequisite for fighting one's way
in a hostile world and for wanting to defeat others in
the fray. In the detached type the spirit is like Robin-
son Crusoe's: he has to be resourceful in order to live.
It is the only way he can compensate for his isolation.

A more precarious way to maintain self-sufficiency
is by consciously or unconsciously restricting one's
needs. We shall better understand the various moves
in this direction if we remember that the underlying
principle here is never to become so attached to anybody or anything that he or it becomes indispensable.

That would jeopardize aloofness. Better to have nothing matter much. For example: A detached person may be capable of real enjoyment, but if enjoyment depends in any way on others he prefers to forego it. He can take pleasure in an occasional evening with a few friends but dislikes general gregariousness and social functions. Similarly, he avoids competition, prestige, and success. He is inclined to restrict his eating, drinking, and living habits and keeps them on a scale that will not require him to spend too much time or energy in earning the money to pay for them. He may bitterly resent illness, considering it a humiliation because it forces him to depend on others. He may insist on acquiring his knowledge of any subject at first hand: rather than take what others have said or written about Russia, for instance, or about this country if he is a foreigner, he will want to see or hear for himself. This attitude would make for splendid inner independence if it were not carried to absurd lengths, like refusing to ask directions when in a strange town.

Another pronounced need is his need for privacy. He is like a person in a hotel room who rarely removes the "Do-Not-Disturb" sign from his door. Even books may be regarded as intruders, as something from outside. Any question put to him about his personal life may shock him; he tends to shroud himself in a veil of secrecy. A patient once told me that at the age of forty-five he still resented the idea of God's omniscience quite as much as when his mother told him that God could look through the shutters and see him biting his fingernails. This was a patient who was extremely reticent about even the most trivial details of his life.

A detached person may be extremely irritated if others take him "for granted"—it makes him feel he is being stepped on. As a rule he prefers to work, sleep, eat alone. In distinct contrast to the compliant type he dislikes sharing any experience—the other person might disturb him. Even when he listens to music, walks or talks with others, his real enjoyment only comes later, in retrospect.

Self-sufficiency and privacy both serve his most outstanding need, the need for utter independence. He himself considers his independence a thing of positive value. And it undoubtedly has a value of sorts. For no matter what his deficiencies, the detached person is certainly no conforming automaton. His refusal blindly to concur, together with his aloofness from competitive struggle, does give him a certain integrity. The fallacy here is that he looks upon independence as an end in itself and ignores the fact that its value depends ultimately upon what he does with it. His independence, like the whole phenomenon of detachment of which it is a part, has a negative orientation; it is aimed at *not* being influenced, coerced, tied, obligated.

Like any other neurotic trend, the need for independence is compulsive and indiscriminate. It manifests itself in a hypersensitivity to everything in any way resembling coercion, influence, obligation, and so on. The degree of sensitivity is a good gauge of the intensity of the detachment. What is felt as constraint varies with the individual. Physical pressure from such things as collars, neckties, girdles, shoes may so be felt. Any obstruction of view may arouse the feeling of being hemmed in; to be in a tunnel or mine may produce anx-

iety. Sensitivity in this direction is not the full explanation of claustrophobia, but it is at any rate its background. Long-term obligations are if possible avoided:
to sign a contract, to sign a lease for more than a year,
to marry are difficult. Marriage for the detached person
is of course a precarious proposition in any event because of the human intimacy involved—although a need
for protection or a belief that the partner will completely fit in with his own peculiarities may mitigate the
risk. Frequently there is an onset of panic before the
consummation of marriage. Time in its inexorableness
is for the most part felt as coercion; the habit of being
just five minutes late on the job may be resorted to in
order to maintain an illusion of freedom. Timetables
constitute a threat; detached patients will enjoy the
story of the man who refused to look at a timetable and
went to the station whenever it happened to suit him,
preferring to wait there for the next train. Other persons' expecting him to do certain things or behave in a
certain way makes him uneasy and rebellious, regardless
of whether such expectations are actually expressed or
merely assumed to exist. For example, he may ordinarily
like to give presents, but will forget about birthday and
Christmas presents because these are expected of him.
To conform with accepted rules of behavior or traditional sets of values is repellent to him. He will conform
outwardly in order to avoid friction, but in his own
mind he stubbornly rejects all conventional rules and
standards. Finally, advice is felt as domination and
meets with resistance even when it coincides with his
own wishes. Resistance in this case may also be linked
with a conscious or unconscious wish to frustrate others.

The need to feel superior, although common to all neuroses, must be stressed here because of its intrinsic association with detachment. The expressions "ivory tower" and "splendid isolation" are evidence that even in common parlance, detachment and superiority are almost invariably linked. Probably nobody can stand isolation without either *being* particularly strong and resourceful or *feeling* uniquely significant. This is corroborated by clinical experience. When the detached person's feeling of superiority is temporarily shattered, whether by a concrete failure or an increase of inner conflicts, he will be unable to stand solitude and may reach out frantically for affection and protection. Vacillations of this kind often appear in his life history. In his teens or early twenties he may have had a few rather lukewarm friendships, but lived on the whole a fairly isolated life, feeling comparatively at ease. He would weave fantasies of a future when he would accomplish exceptional things. But later these dreams were shipwrecked on the rocks of reality. Though in high school he had had undisputed claim to first place, in college he ran up against serious competition and recoiled from it. His first attempts at love relationships failed. Or he realized as he grew older that his dreams were not materializing. Aloofness then became unbearable and he was consumed by a compulsive drive for human intimacy, for sexual relations, for marriage. He was willing to submit to any indignity, if only he were loved. When such a person comes for analytical treatment, his detachment, though still pronounced and obvious, cannot be tackled. All he wants at first is help to find love in one form or another. Only when he feels considerably stronger does he discover with immense relief that he would much rather "live alone and like it." The impression is that he has merely reverted to his former detachment. But actually it is a matter of being now for the first time on solid enough ground to admit— even to himself—that isolation is what he wants. This would be the appropriate time to work on his detachment.

The need for superiority in the case of the detached person has certain specific features. Abhorring competitive struggle, he does not want to excel realistically through consistent effort. He feels rather that the treasures within him should be recognized without any effort on his part; his hidden greatness should be felt without his having to make a move. In his dreams, for instance, he may picture stores of treasure hidden away in some remote village which connoisseurs come from far to see. Like all notions of superiority this contains an element of reality. The hidden treasure symbolizes his intellectual and emotional life which he guards within the magic circle.

Another way his sense of superiority expresses itself is in his feeling of his own uniqueness. This is a direct outgrowth of his wanting to feel separate and distinct from others. He may liken himself to a tree standing alone on a hilltop, while the trees in the forest below are stunted by those about them. Where the compliant type looks at his fellow man with the silent question, "Will he like me?"—and the aggressive type wants to know, "How strong an adversary is he?" or "Can he be useful to me?"—the detached person's first concern is, "Will he interfere with me? Will he want to influence

me or will he leave me alone?" The scene in which
Peer Gynt meets the buttonmolder is a perfect symbolic
representation of the terror the detached person feels
at being thrown with others. His own room in hell
would be all right, but to be tossed into a melting pot,
to be molded or adapted to others, is a horrifying
thought. He feels himself akin to a rare oriental rug,
unique in its pattern and combination of colors, forever
unalterable. He takes extraordinary pride in having
kept free of the leveling influences of environment and
is determined to keep on doing so. In cherishing his
unchangeableness he raises the rigidity inherent in all
neuroses to the dignity of a sacred principle. Willing
and even eager to elaborate his own pattern, to give it
greater purity and lucidity, he insists that nothing ex-
trinsic be injected. In all its simplicity and inadequacy
the Peer Gynt maxim stands: "To thyself be enough."

The emotional life of the detached person does not
follow as strict a pattern as that of the other types described. Individual variations are greater in his case,
chiefly because in contradistinction to the other two,
whose predominant trends are directed toward positive
goals—affection, intimacy, love in the one; survival,
domination, success in the other—his goals are negative:
he wants *not* to be involved, *not* to need anybody, *not*
to allow others to intrude on or influence him. Hence
the emotional picture would be dependent on the particular desires that have developed or been allowed to
stay alive within this negative framework, and only a
limited number of tendencies intrinsic to detachment
as such can be formulated.

There is a general tendency to suppress all feeling, even to deny its existence. I should like to quote here a passage from an unpublished novel of the poet Anna Maria Armi, because it succinctly expresses not only this tendency but also other typical attitudes of the detached person. The main character, reminiscing about his adolescence, says: "I could visualize a strong physical tie (as I had with my father) and a strong spiritual tie (as I had with my heroes), but I could not see where or how feeling came into it; feelings simply didn't exist —people lied about that as about so many other things. B. was horrified. 'But how do you explain sacrifice?' she said. For a moment I was astounded by the truth in her remark; then I decided that sacrifice was just another of the lies, and when it was not a lie it was either a physical or spiritual act. I dreamed at that time of living alone, of never marrying, of becoming strong and peaceful without talking too much, without asking for help. I wanted to work on myself, to be freer and freer, to give up dreams in order to see and live clearly. I thought morals had no meaning; being good or bad made no difference as long as you were absolutely true. The great sin was to look for sympathy or to expect help. Souls seemed to me temples that had to be guarded, and inside them there were always strange ceremonies going on, known only to their priests, their custodians."

The rejection of feeling pertains primarily to feelings toward other people and applies to both love and hate. It is a logical consequence of the need to keep at an emotional distance from others, in that strong love or hate, consciously experienced, would bring one either close to others or into conflict with them. H. S. Sullivan's term, distance machinery, is appropriate here. It does not necessarily follow that feeling will be suppressed in areas outside human relationships and become active in the realm of books, animals, nature, art, food, and so on. But there is considerable danger of this. For a person capable of deep and passionate emotion it may be impossible to suppress only one sector of his feelings —and that the most crucial—without going the whole length of suppressing feeling altogether. This is speculative reasoning, but certainly the following is true. Artists of the detached type, who have demonstrated in their creative periods that they can not only feel deeply but also give expression to it, have often gone through periods, usually in adolescence, of either complete emotional numbness or of vigorous denial of all feeling—as in the passage quoted. The creative periods seem to occur when, following some disastrous attempts at close relationships, they have either deliberately or spontaneously adapted their lives to detachment—that is, when they have consciously or unconsciously determined to keep at a distance from others, or have become resigned to a kind of isolated living. The fact that now, at a safe distance from others, they can release and express a host of feelings not directly connected with human relationships permits the interpretation that the early denial of all feeling was necessary to the achievement of their detachment.

Another reason why the suppression of feeling may go beyond the sphere of human relationships has already been suggested in our discussion of self-sufficiency. Any desire, interest, or enjoyment that might make the detached person dependent upon others is viewed as treachery from within and may be checked on that account. It is as if every situation had to be carefully tested from the standpoint of a possible loss of freedom before feeling could be allowed full play. Any threat of dependence will cause him to withdraw emotionally. But when he finds a situation quite safe in this regard he can enjoy it to the full. Thoreau's *Walden* is a good illustration of the profound emotional experience possible under these conditions. The lurking fear of either becoming too attached to a pleasure or of its infringing upon his freedom indirectly will sometimes make him verge on the ascetic. But it is an asceticism of its own kind—not oriented toward self-denial or self-torture. We might rather call it a self-discipline which—accepting the premises—is not lacking in wisdom.

It is of great importance to psychic balance that there be areas accessible to spontaneous emotional experience. Creative abilities, for instance, may be a kind of salvation. If their expression has been inhibited, and if then through analysis or some other experience it is liberated, the beneficent effect upon the detached person can be so great as to make it look like a miraculous cure. Caution is in order in evaluating such cures. In the first place it would be a mistake to make any generalization about their occurrence: what may mean salvation for a detached person will not necessarily have any such meaning for others.[1] And even for him it is

[1] *Cf.* Daniel Schneider, "The Motion of the Neurotic Pattern; Its Distortion of Creative Mastery and Sexual Power." Paper read before the Academy of Medicine, May 26, 1943.

not strictly a "cure" in the sense of a radical change in neurotic fundamentals. It merely allows him a more satisfactory and less disturbed way of living.

The more the emotions are checked, the more likely it is that emphasis will be placed upon intelligence. The expectation then will be that everything can be solved by sheer power of reasoning, as if mere knowledge of one's own problems would be sufficient to cure them. Or as if reasoning alone could cure all the troubles of the world!

In view of all we have said about the detached person's human relationships it will be clear that any close and lasting relation would be bound to jeopardize his detachment and hence would be likely to be disastrous—unless the partner should be equally detached and so of his own accord respect the need for distance, or unless he is able and willing for other reasons to adapt himself to such needs. A Solveig who in loving devotion patiently awaits Peer Gynt's return is the ideal partner. Solveig expects nothing from him. Expectations on her part would frighten him as much as would loss of control over his own feelings. Mostly he is unaware of how little he himself gives, and he believes he has bestowed his unexpressed and unlived feelings, so precious to himself, upon the partner. Provided emotional distance is sufficiently guaranteed, he may be able to preserve a considerable measure of enduring loyalty. He may be capable of having intense short-lived relationships, relationships in which he appears and vanishes. They are brittle, and any number of factors may hasten his withdrawal.

Sexual relationships may mean inordinately much to

him as a bridge to others. He will enjoy them if they are transitory and do not interfere with his life. They should be confined, as it were, to the compartment set aside for such affairs. On the other hand he may have cultivated indifference to so great a degree that it permits of no trespassing. Then wholly imaginary relationships may be substituted for real ones.

All the peculiarities we have described appear in the analytical process. Naturally, the detached person resents analysis because indeed it is the greatest possible intrusion upon his private life. But he is also interested in observing himself and may be fascinated by the greater vista it opens upon the intricate processes going on within him. He may be intrigued by the artistic quality of dreams or by the aptness of his inadvertent associations. His joy in finding confirmation for assumptions resembles the scientist's. He is appreciative of the analyst's attention and of his pointing to something here and there, but abominates being urged or "forced" in a direction he has not foreseen. He will often mention the danger of suggestion in analysis—although factually there is less danger of this in his case than for any other type, because he is fully armed against "influence." Far from defending his position in a rational way by testing out the analyst's suggestions, he tends, as is his wont, to reject blindly, though indirectly and politely, all that does not fit in with his own ideas about himself and life in general. He finds it particularly obnoxious that the analyst should expect him to change in any way. Of course he wants to get rid of whatever is disturbing him; but it must not involve a change in his personality. He is almost as unfailingly willing to

observe as he is unconsciously determined to remain
as he is. His defiance of all influence is only one of the
explanations for his attitude, and not the deepest one;
we shall become acquainted with others later on. Naturally he puts a great distance between himself and the
analyst. For a long time the analyst will be only a voice.
In dreams the analytical situation may appear as a long-
distance call between two reporters on different conti-
nents. At first glance a dream like this would seem to
express the remoteness he feels toward the analyst and
the analytical process—merely an accurate presentation
of an attitude that exists consciously. But since dreams
are a search for a solution rather than a mere description of existing feelings, the deeper meaning of such
a dream is a *wish* to keep his relationship to the analyst
and to the whole analytical process away from him—
not to let the analysis touch him in any way.

A final characteristic observable both in the analysis
and outside it is the tremendous vigor with which the
detachment is defended when attacked. The same might
be said of every neurotic position. But the fight in this
case seems to be more tenacious, almost a life and death
struggle for which all available resources must be mobi-
lized. The battle really starts in a quiet subversive way
long before the detachment is attacked. Keeping the
analyst out of the picture is one phase of it. If the
analyst tries to convince the patient that there is some
relationship between them and that something is likely
to go on in the patient's mind on this score, he meets
with a more or less elaborate, courteous repudiation.
At best the patient will express some rational thoughts
he has had about the analyst. If a spontaneous emo-

tional reaction should appear he will not pursue it further. In addition, there is frequently a deep-seated resistance to having anything pertaining to human relationships analyzed. The patient's relations to others are kept so vague that it is often difficult for the analyst to get any clear picture of them. And this reluctance is understandable. He has preserved a safe distance from others; talking about the matter could only prove disturbing, upsetting. Repeated attempts to pursue the subject may be met with open suspicion. Does the analyst want to make the patient gregarious? (For him this is beneath contempt.) If at a later period the analyst succeeds in showing him some definite drawbacks to detachment, the patient becomes frightened and irritable. He may think at this point of quitting. Outside analysis his reactions are if anything still more violent. These ordinarily quiet and rational persons may freeze with rage or become actually abusive if their aloofness and independence are threatened. Positive panic may be induced at the thought of joining any movement or professional group where real participation and not merely payment of dues is required. If they do become involved they may thrash about blindly to extricate themselves. They can be more expert in finding methods of escape than a man whose life is attacked. Were the choice between love and independence, as a patient once put it, they would choose independence without hesitation. This brings up another point. Not only are they willing to defend their detachment by every available means, but they find no sacrifice too great in its behalf. External advantages and inner values will be equally renounced—consciously, by setting aside any desire that might interfere with independence, or unconsciously, by automatic prohibition.

Anything so vigorously defended must have an overwhelming subjective value. We can hope to understand the functions of detachment and eventually to be helpful therapeutically only if we are aware of this. As we have seen, each of the basic attitudes toward others has its positive value. In moving toward people the person tries to create for himself a friendly relation to his world. In moving against people he equips himself for survival in a competitive society. In moving away from people he hopes to attain a certain integrity and serenity. As a matter of fact, all three attitudes are not only desirable but necessary to our development as human beings. It is only when they appear and operate in a neurotic framework that they become compulsive, rigid, indiscriminate, and mutually exclusive. This considerably detracts from their value, but does not destroy it.

The gains to be derived from detachment are indeed considerable. It is significant that in all oriental philosophies detachment is sought as a basis for high spiritual development. Of course we cannot compare such aspirations with those of neurotic detachment. There detachment is voluntarily chosen as the best approach to self-fulfillment and is adopted by persons who could, if they wanted, live a different kind of life; neurotic detachment, on the other hand, is not a matter of choice but of inner compulsion, the only possible way of living. Nonetheless, some of the same benefits may be derived from it—though the extent to which this will be so depends on the severity of the whole neurotic process. In spite of the ravaging force of a neurosis, the detached person may preserve a certain integrity. This would hardly be a factor in a society in which human relationships were generally friendly and honest. But in a society in which there is much hypocrisy, crookedness, envy, cruelty and greed, the integrity of a none too strong person easily suffers; keeping at a distance helps to maintain it. Furthermore, since neurosis usually robs a person of his peace of mind, detachment may provide an avenue of serenity, its extent varying with the amount of sacrifice he is willing to make. Detachment allows him, in addition, some measure of original thinking and feeling, provided that within his magic circle emotional life has not been altogether deadened. Lastly, all of these factors, together with his contemplative relation to the world and the comparative absence of distraction, contribute toward the development and expression of creative abilities, if he has any. I do not mean that neurotic detachment is a precondition for creation, but that under neurotic stress detachment will provide the best chance of expressing what creative ability there is.

Substantial though these gains may be, they do not seem to be the main reason why detachment is so desperately defended. Actually the defense is equally desperate if for one reason or another the gains are minimal or are heavily overshadowed by concomitant disturbances. This observation leads into further depths. If the detached person is thrown into close contact with others he may very readily go to pieces or, to use the popular term, have a nervous breakdown. I use the term advisedly here because it covers a wide range of disturbances—functional disorders, alcoholism, suicidal attempts, depression, incapacity for work, psychotic episodes. The patient himself, and sometimes the psychiatrist too, tends to relate the disturbance to some upsetting event that occurred just prior to the "breakdown." A sergeant's unjust discrimination, a husband's philandering and lying about it, a wife's behaving neurotically, a homosexual episode, unpopularity in college, the need to make a living when life has previously been sheltered, and so on may be held to blame. True enough any such problem is relevant. The therapist should take it seriously and try to understand what in particular was set off in the patient by a specific difficulty. But to do that is hardly sufficient, because the question remains why the patient has been so intensely affected, why his whole psychic equilibrium has been endangered by a difficulty which by and large cannot be considered greater than ordinary frustrations and upsets. In other words, even when the analyst understands how the patient reacted to a particular difficulty, he still needs to understand why there is such a distinct disproportion between the provocation and its effect.

In answer we could point to the fact that the neurotic trends involved in detachment, like other neurotic trends, give the individual a feeling of security as long as they function, and that, conversely, anxiety is aroused when they fail to function. As long as the detached person can keep at a distance he feels comparatively safe; if for any reason the magic circle is penetrated, his security is threatened. This consideration brings us closer to an understanding of why the detached person becomes panicky if he can no longer safeguard his emotional distance from others—and we should add that the reason his panic is so great is that he has no technique for dealing with life. He can only keep aloof and avoid life, as it were. Here again it is the negative quality of detachment that gives the picture a special color, different from that of other neurotic trends. To be more specific, in a difficult situation the detached person can neither appease nor fight, neither co-operate nor dictate terms, neither love nor be ruthless. He is as defenseless as an animal that has only one means of coping with danger—that is, to escape and hide. Appropriating pictures and analogies that have appeared in associations or dreams: he is like the pygmies of Ceylon, invincible so long as they hide in the forests but easily beaten when they emerge. He is like a medieval town protected by one wall only—if that wall is taken, the town is defenseless against the enemy. Such a position fully justifies his anxiety toward life in general. It helps us to understand his remoteness as an over-all protection to which he must tenaciously cling and which he must defend at whatever cost. All neurotic trends are at bottom defensive moves, but the others also constitute an attempt to cope with life in a positive way. When detachment is the predominant trend it renders a person so helpless in any realistic dealing with life that in the course of time its defensive character becomes uppermost.

But the desperateness with which detachment is defended has a further explanation. The threat to detachment, "smashing the wall," often means more than temporary panic. What may result is a kind of disintegration of personality in psychotic episodes. If in anal-

ysis detachment begins to crumble, the patient not only
becomes diffusely apprehensive but directly and indirectly expresses definite fears. There may be, for instance, a fear of becoming submerged in the amorphous
mass of human beings, a fear, primarily, of losing his
uniqueness. There is also the fear of being helplessly
exposed to the coercion and exploitation of aggressive
persons—a result of his utter defenselessness. But there
is still a third fear, that of going insane, which may
emerge so vividly that the patient wants positive reassurance against such a possibility. Going insane in this context does not mean going berserk, nor is it a reaction to
an emerging wish for irresponsibility. It is a straight expression of the specific fear of being split right open,
often expressed in dreams and associations. This would
suggest that relinquishing his detachment would bring
him face to face with his own conflicts; that he would
not be able to survive it but would be split like a tree
struck by lightning, to use an image that occurred to a
patient. This assumption is confirmed by other observa-
tions. Highly detached persons have an almost insurmountable aversion to the idea of inner conflicts. Later
they will tell the analyst that they simply didn't know
what he was talking about when he spoke of conflicts.
Whenever the analyst succeeds in showing them a conflict operating within themselves, they will imperceptibly and with amazing unconscious skill veer away from
the subject. If, inadvertently, before they are ready to
admit it, they recognize a conflict in a momentary flash,
they are seized with acute panic. When later they approach the recognition of conflicts on a more secure
basis, a greater wave of detachment follows.

Thus we arrive at a conclusion that at first glance would have been bewildering. Detachment is an intrinsic part of the basic conflict, but it is also a protection against it. The puzzle resolves itself, however, if we are more specific. It is a protection against the two more active partners in the basic conflict. Here we must reiterate the statement that the predominance of one of the basic attitudes does not prevent the other contradictory ones from existing and operating. We can see this play of forces in the detached personality even more clearly than in the other two groups described. To begin with, the contradictory strivings often show in the life history. Before he has clearly accepted his detachment a person of this type will often have gone through episodes of compliance and dependence as well as through periods of aggressive and ruthless rebellion. In contrast to the clearly defined values of the other two types, his sets of values are most contradictory. In addition to his permanent high evaluation of what he regards as freedom and independence, he may at some time in the analysis express an extreme appreciation for human goodness, sympathy, generosity, self-effacing sacrifice, and at another time swing to a complete jungle philosophy of callous self-interest. He himself may feel puzzled by these contradictions, but with some rationalization or other he will try to deny their conflicting character. The analyst will easily become confused if he has no clear perspective of the whole structure. He may try to follow one path or the other without getting very far in either direction because again and again the patient takes refuge in his detachment, thereby shutting all the gateways as one would shut the watertight bulkheads of a ship.

There is a perfect and simple logic underlying the special "resistance" of the detached person. He does not want to relate himself to the analyst or to take cognizance of him as a human being. He does not really want to analyze his human relationships at all. He does not want to face his conflicts. And if we understand his premise, we see that he cannot even be interested in analyzing any of these factors. His premise is the conscious conviction that he need not bother about his relations with others so long as he keeps at a safe distance from them; that a disturbance in these relations will not upset him if only he keeps away from others; that even the conflicts of which the analyst speaks can and should be left dormant because they will only bother him; and that there is no need to straighten things out because he will not budge from his detachment anyway. As we have said, this unconscious reasoning is logically correct—up to a point. What he leaves out and for a long time refuses to recognize is that he cannot possibly grow and develop in a vacuum.

The all-important function of neurotic detachment, then, is to keep major conflicts out of operation. It is the most radical and most effective of the defenses erected against them. One of the many neurotic ways of creating an artificial harmony, it is an attempt at solution through evasion. But it is no true solution because the compulsive cravings for closeness as well as for aggressive domination, exploitation, and excelling remain, and they keep harassing if not paralyzing their carrier. Finally, no real inner peace or freedom can ever be attained as long as the contradictory sets of values continue to exist.

CHAPTER SIX

The Idealized Image

OUR DISCUSSION of the neurotic's fundamental attitudes toward others has acquainted us with two of the major ways in which he attempts to solve his conflicts or, more precisely, to dispose of them. One of these consists in repressing certain aspects of the personality and bringing their opposites to the fore; the other is to put such distance between oneself and one's fellows that the conflicts are set out of operation. Both processes induce a feeling of unity that permits the individual to function, even if at considerable cost to himself.[1]

A further attempt, here to be described, is the creation of an image of what the neurotic believes himself to be, or of what at the time he feels he can or ought to be. Conscious or unconscious, the image is always in large degree removed from reality, though the influence it exerts on the person's life is very real indeed. What is more, it is always flattering in character, as illustrated by a cartoon in the *New Yorker* in which a large middle-aged woman sees herself in the mirror a slender young girl. The particular features of the image vary and are determined by the structure of the personality: beauty may be held to be outstanding, or power,

[1] Herman Nunberg dealt with this problem of the striving for unity in his paper, "Die Synthetische Funktion des Ich," *Internationale Zeitschrift für Psychoanalyse*, 1930.

intelligence, genius, saintliness, honesty, or what you will. Precisely to the extent that the image is unrealistic, it tends to make the person arrogant, in the original meaning of the word; for arrogance, though used synonymously with superciliousness, means to arrogate to oneself qualities that one does not have, or that one has potentially but not factually. And the more unrealistic the image, the more it makes the person vulnerable and avid for outside affirmation and recognition. We do not need confirmation for qualities of which we are certain, but we will be extremely touchy when false claims are questioned.

We can observe this idealized image at its most blatant in the grandiose notions of psychotics; but in principle its characteristics are the same in neurotics. It is less fantastic here, but it may be just as real to them. If we regard the degree of removal from reality as marking the difference between psychoses and neuroses, we may consider the idealized image as a bit of psychosis woven into the texture of neurosis.

In all its essentials the idealized image is an unconscious phenomenon. Although his self-inflation may be most obvious even to an untrained observer, the neurotic is not aware that he is idealizing himself. Nor does he know what a bizarre conglomeration of characters is assembled here. He may have a vague sense that he is making high demands upon himself, but mistaking such perfectionist demands for genuine ideals he in no way questions their validity and is indeed rather proud of them.

How his creation affects his attitude toward himself

varies with the individual and depends largely on the focus of interest. If the neurotic's interest lies in convincing himself that he *is* his idealized image, he develops the belief that he is in fact the mastermind, the exquisite human being, whose very faults are divine.[2] If the focus is on the realistic self which by comparison with the idealized image is highly despicable, self-derogatory criticism is in the foreground. Since the picture of the self that results from such disparagement is just as far removed from reality as is the idealized image, it could appropriately be called the despised image. If, finally, the focus is upon the discrepancy between the idealized image and the actual self, then all he is aware of and all we can observe are his incessant attempts to bridge the gap and whip himself into perfection. In this event he keeps reiterating the word "should" with amazing frequency. He keeps telling us what he should have felt, thought, done. He is at bottom as convinced of his inherent perfection as the naïvely "narcissistic" person, and betrays it by the belief that he actually could be perfect if only he were more strict with himself, more controlled, more alert, more circumspect.

In contrast to authentic ideals, the idealized image has a static quality. It is not a goal toward whose attainment he strives but a fixed idea which he worships. Ideals have a dynamic quality; they arouse an incentive to approximate them; they are an indispensable and invaluable force for growth and development. The ideal-

[2] *Cf.* Anne Parrish, "All Kneeling," *The Second Woollcott Reader,* Garden City Publishing Co., 1939.

ized image is a decided hindrance to growth because it
either denies shortcomings or merely condemns them.
Genuine ideals make for humility, the idealized image
for arrogance.

This phenomenon—however defined—has long been
recognized. It is referred to in the philosophic writings
of all times. Freud introduced it into the theory of
neurosis, calling it by a variety of names: ego ideal,
narcissism, superego. It forms the central thesis of
Adler's psychology, described there as a striving for
superiority. It would lead us too far afield to point out
in detail the differences and similarities between these
concepts and my own.[3] Briefly, all of these are concerned only with one or another aspect of the idealized
image, and fail to see the phenomenon as a whole.
Hence despite pertinent comment and argument not
only by Freud and Adler but by many other writers
as well—among them Franz Alexander, Paul Federn,
Bernard Glueck, and Ernest Jones—the full significance
of the phenomenon and its functions has not been recognized. What, then, are its functions? Apparently it
fulfills vital needs. No matter how the various writers
account for it theoretically, they are all agreed on the
one point that it constitutes a stronghold of neurosis
difficult to shake or even to weaken. Freud for one regarded a deeply ingrained "narcissistic" attitude as
among the most serious obstacles to therapy.

[3] *Cf.* the critical examination of Freud's concept of narcissism,
superego, and guilt feelings in Karen Horney, *New Ways in
Psychoanalysis,* W. W. Norton, 1938; *cf. also* Erich Fromm, "Self-
ishness and Self-Love," *Psychiatry,* 1939.

To begin with what is perhaps its most elementary function, the idealized image substitutes for realistic self-confidence and realistic pride. A person who eventually becomes neurotic has little chance to build up initial self-confidence because of the crushing experiences he has been subjected to. Such self-confidence as he may have is further weakened in the course of his neurotic development because the very conditions indispensable for self-confidence are apt to be destroyed. It is difficult to formulate these conditions briefly. The most important factors are the aliveness and availability of one's emotional energies, the development of authentic goals of one's own, and the faculty of being an active instrument in one's own life. However a neurosis develops, just these things are liable to be damaged. Neurotic trends impair self-determination because a person is then driven instead of being himself the driver. Moreover, the neurotic's capacity to determine his own paths is continually weakened by his dependence upon people, whatever form this may have assumed—blind rebellion, blind craving to excel, and a blind need to keep away from others are all forms of dependence. Further, by inhibiting great sectors of emotional energy, he puts them completely out of action. All of these factors make it nearly impossible for him to develop his own goals. Last but not least, the basic conflict makes him divided in his own house. Being thus deprived of a substantial foundation, the neurotic must inflate his feeling of significance and power. That is why a belief in his omnipotence is a never-failing component of the idealized image.

A second function is closely linked with the first. The neurotic does not feel weak in a vacuum but in a world peopled with enemies ready to cheat, humiliate, enslave, and defeat him. He must therefore constantly measure and compare himself with others, not for reasons of vanity or caprice but by bitter necessity. And since at bottom he feels weak and contemptible—as we shall see later on—he must search for something that will make him feel better, more worthy than others. Whether it takes the form of feeling more saintly or more ruthless, more loving or more cynical, he must in his own mind feel superior in some way—regardless of any particular drive to excel. For the most part such a need contains elements of wanting to triumph over others, because no matter what the structure of the neurosis there is always vulnerability and a readiness to feel looked down on and humiliated. The need for vindictive triumph as an antidote to feeling humiliated may be acted upon or may exist mainly in the neurotic's own mind; it may be conscious or unconscious, but it is one of the driving forces in the neurotic need for superiority and gives it its special coloring.[4] The competitive spirit of this civilization is not only conducive to fostering neuroses in general, through the disturbances in human relationships it creates, but it also specifically feeds this need for pre-eminence.

We have seen how the idealized image substitutes for true self-confidence and pride. But there is yet another way in which it serves as surrogate. Since the neurotic's ideals are contradictory they cannot possibly have any

[4] *Cf.* Chapter 12, Sadistic Trends.

obligating power; remaining dim and undefined, they can give him no guidance. Hence if it were not that his endeavor to be his self-created idol gave a kind of meaning to his life he would feel wholly without purpose. This becomes particularly apparent in the course of analysis, when the undermining of his idealized image gives him for a time the feeling of being quite lost. And it is only then that he recognizes his confusion in the matter of ideals and that this begins to strike him as undesirable. Before, the whole subject was beyond his understanding and interest, no matter how much lip service he gave it; now for the first time he realizes that ideals have some meaning, and wants to discover what his own ideals really are. This kind of experience is evidence, I should say, that the idealized image substitutes for genuine ideals. An understanding of this function has significance for therapy. The analyst may point out to the patient at an earlier period the contradictions in his set of values. But he cannot expect any constructive interest in the subject and hence cannot work on it until the idealized image has become dispensable.

To a greater degree than any of the others, one particular function of the image can be held accountable for its rigidity. If in our private mirror we see ourselves as paragons of virtue or intelligence, even our most blatant faults and handicaps will disappear or acquire attractive coloration—just as in a good painting a shabby, decaying wall is no longer a shabby, decaying wall but a beautiful composite of brown and gray and reddish color values.

We can arrive at a deeper understanding of this defensive function if we raise the simple question: What does a person regard as his faults and shortcomings? It is one of those questions that at first sight does not seem to lead anywhere because one starts to think of infinite possibilities. Nevertheless there is a fairly concrete answer. What a person regards as his faults and shortcomings depends on what he accepts or rejects in himself. That, however—under similar cultural conditions—is determined by which aspect of the basic conflict predominates. The compliant type, for instance, does not regard his fears or his helplessness as a taint, whereas the aggressive type would regard any such feeling as shameful, to be hidden from oneself and others. The compliant type registers his hostile aggressions as sinful; the aggressive type looks upon his softer feelings as contemptible weakness. Each type, in addition, is driven to reject all that is actually mere pretense on the part of his more acceptable self. The compliant type, for instance, has to reject the fact that he is not a genuinely loving and generous person; the detached type does not want to see that his aloofness is not a matter of his own free choice, that he must keep apart because he cannot cope with others, and so on. Both, as a rule, reject sadistic trends (to be discussed later). We would thus arrive at the conclusion that what is regarded as a shortcoming and rejected is whatever does not fit into the consistent picture created by the predominant attitude toward others. And we could say that the defensive function of the idealized image is to negate the existence of conflicts; that is why it must of necessity remain so immovable. Before I recognized this I often wondered why it is so impossible for a patient to accept himself as a little less significant, a little less superior. But looked at this way the answer is clear. He cannot budge an inch because the recognition of certain short-comings would confront him with his conflicts, thus jeopardizing the artificial harmony he has established. We can arrive, therefore, at a positive correlation between the intensity of the conflicts and the rigidity of the idealized image: an especially elaborate and rigid image permits us to infer especially disruptive conflicts.

Over and above the four functions already pointed out, the idealized image has still a fifth, likewise related to the basic conflict. The image has a more positive use than merely to camouflage the conflict's unacceptable parts. It represents a kind of artistic creation in which opposites appear reconciled or in which, at any rate, they no longer appear as conflicts to the individual himself. A few examples will show how this happens. In order to avoid lengthy reports I shall merely name the conflicts present and show how they appeared in the idealized image.

The predominating aspect of X's conflict was compliance—a great need for affection and approval, to be taken care of, to be sympathetic, generous, considerate, loving. Second in prominence was detachment, with the usual aversion to joining groups, emphasis on independence, fear of ties, sensitivity to coercion. The detachment constantly clashed with the need for human intimacy and created repeated disturbances in his relations with women. Aggressive drives, too, were quite apparent, manifesting themselves in his having to be first in any situation, in dominating others indirectly, occasionally exploiting them, and tolerating no interference. Naturally these tendencies detracted considerably from his capacity for love and friendship, and clashed as well with his detachment. Unaware of these drives, he had fabricated an idealized image that was a composite of three figures. He was the great lover and friend—incredible that any woman could care more for another man; nobody was so kind and good as he. He was the greatest leader of his time, a political genius held much in awe. And finally he was the great philosopher, the man of wisdom, one of the few gifted with profound insight into the meaning of life and its ultimate futility.

The image was not altogether fantastic. He had ample potentialities in all these directions. But the potentialities had been raised to the level of accomplished fact, of great and unique achievement. Moreover, the compulsive nature of the drives had been obscured and was replaced by a belief in innate qualities and gifts. Instead of a neurotic need for affection and approval there was a supposed capacity to love; instead of a drive to excel, assumed superior gifts; instead of a need for aloofness, independence and wisdom. Finally and most important, the conflicts were exorcised in the following way. The drives which in real life interfered with one another and prevented him from fulfilling any of his potentialities were promoted to the realm of abstract perfection, appearing as several compatible aspects of a rich personality; and the three aspects of the basic conflict which they represented were isolated in the three figures that made up his idealized image.

Another example brings into clearer relief the importance of isolating the conflicting elements.[5] In the case of Y the predominant trend was detachment, in a rather extreme form, with all the implications described in the previous chapter. His tendency to comply was also quite marked, though Y himself shut it out from awareness because it was too incompatible with his desire for independence. Strivings to be extremely good occasionally broke forcibly through the shell of repression. A longing for human intimacy was conscious, and clashed continuously with his detachment. He could be ruthlessly aggressive only in his imagination: he indulged in fantasies of mass destruction, wishing quite frankly to kill all those who interfered with his life; he professed to believe in a jungle philosophy—the gospel of might makes right, with its ruthless pursuit of self-interest, was the only intelligent and unhypocritical way of living. In his actual living, however, he was rather timid; explosions of violence occurred under certain conditions only.

His idealized image was the following odd combination. Most of the time he was a hermit living on a mountaintop, having attained to infinite wisdom and serenity. At rare intervals he could turn into a werewolf, entirely devoid of human feelings, bent on killing. And as if

[5] In that classic illustration of dual personality, Robert Louis Stevenson's *Dr. Jekyll and Mr. Hyde,* the main idea is built around the possibility of separating the conflicting elements in man. After recognizing how radical is the schism between good and evil within himself, Dr. Jekyll says: "From an early date . . . I had learned to dwell with pleasure, as a beloved daydream, on the thought of the separation of these elements. If each, I told myself, could but be housed in separate identities, life would be relieved of all that was unbearable."

these two incompatible figures were not enough, he was as well the ideal friend and lover.

We see here the same denial of neurotic trends, the same self-aggrandizement, the same mistaking of potentialities for realities. In this instance, though, no attempt has been made to reconcile the conflicts; the contradictions remain. But—in contrast to real life—they appear pure and undiluted. Because they are isolated they do not interfere with one another. And that seems to be what counts. The conflicts as such have disappeared.

One last example of a more unified idealized image: In the factual behavior of Z aggressive trends strongly predominated, accompanied by sadistic tendencies. He was domineering and inclined to exploit. Driven by a devouring ambition, he pushed ruthlessly ahead. He could plan, organize, fight, and adhered consciously to an unmitigated jungle philosophy. He was also extremely detached; but since his aggressive drives always entangled him with groups of people, he could not maintain his aloofness. He kept strict guard, though, not to get involved in any personal relationship nor to let himself enjoy anything to which people were essential contributors. In this he succeeded fairly well, because positive feelings for others were greatly repressed; desires for human intimacy were mainly channeled along sexual lines. There was present, however, a distinct tendency to comply, together with a need for approval that interfered with his craving for power. And there were underlying puritanical standards, used chiefly as a whip over others—but which of course he could not help applying to himself as well—that clashed head-long with his jungle philosophy.

In his idealized image he was the knight in shining armor, the crusader with wide and unfailing vision, ever pursuing the right. As becomes a wise leader, he was not personally attached to anyone but dispensed a stern though just discipline. He was honest without being hypocritical. Women loved him and he could be a great lover but was not tied to any woman. Here the same goal is achieved as in the other instances: the elements of the basic conflict are blended.

The idealized image is thus an attempt at solving the basic conflict, an attempt of at least as great importance as the others I have described. It has the enormous subjective value of serving as a binder, of holding together a divided individual. And although it exists only in the person's mind, it exerts a decisive influence on his relations with others.

The idealized image might be called a fictitious or illusory self, but that would be only a half truth and hence misleading. The wishful thinking operating in its creation is certainly striking, particularly since it occurs in persons who otherwise stand on a ground of firm reality. But this does not make it wholly fictitious. It is an imaginative creation interwoven with and determined by very realistic factors. It usually contains traces of the person's genuine ideals. While the grandiose achievements are illusory, the potentialities underlying them are often real. More relevant, it is born of very real inner necessities, it fulfills very real functions, and it has a very real influence on its creator. The processes operating in its creation are determined by such definite laws that a knowledge of its specific features permits us to make accurate inferences as to the true character structure of the particular person.

But regardless of how much fantasy is woven into the idealized image, for the neurotic himself it has the value of reality. The more firmly it is established the more he *is* his idealized image, while his real self is proportionately dimmed out. This reversal of the actual picture is bound to come about because of the very nature of the functions the image performs. Every one of them is aimed at effacing the real personality and turning the spotlight on itself. Looking back over the history of many patients we are led to believe that its establishment has often been literally lifesaving, and that is why the resistance a patient puts up if his image is attacked is entirely justified, or at least logical. As long as his image remains real to him and is intact, he can feel significant, superior, and harmonious, in spite of the illusory nature of those feelings. He can consider himself entitled to raise all kinds of demands and claims on the basis of his assumed superiority. But if he allows it to be undermined he is immediately threatened with the prospect of facing all his weaknesses, with no title to special claims, a comparatively insignificant figure or even—in his own eyes—a contemptible one. More terrifying still, he is faced with his conflicts and the hideous fear of being torn to pieces. That this may give him a chance of becoming a much better human being, worth more than all the glory of his idealized image, is a gospel he hears but that for a long time means nothing to him. It is a leap in the dark of which he is afraid.

With so great a subjective value to recommend it, the position of the image would be unassailable if it were not for the huge drawbacks inseparable from it. The whole edifice is in the first place extremely rickety by reason of the fictitious elements involved. A treasure house loaded with dynamite, it makes the individual highly vulnerable. Any questioning or criticism from outside, any awareness of his own failure to measure up to the image, any real insight into the forces operating within him can make it explode or crumble. He must restrict his life lest he be exposed to such dangers. He must avoid situations in which he would not be admired or recognized. He must avoid tasks that he is not certain to master. He may even develop an intense aversion to effort of any kind. To him, the gifted one, the mere vision of a picture he might paint is already the master painting. Any mediocre person can get somewhere by hard work; for him to apply himself like every Tom, Dick, and Harry would be an admission that he is not the mastermind, and so humiliating. Since nothing can actually be achieved without work, he defeats by his attitude the very ends he is driven to attain. And the gap between his idealized image and his real self widens.

He is dependent upon endless affirmation from others in the form of approval, admiration, flattery—none of which, however, can give him any more than temporary reassurance. He may unconsciously hate everyone who is overbearing or who, being better than he in any way—more assertive, more evenly balanced, better informed—threatens to undermine his own notions of himself. The more desperately he clings to the belief that he is his idealized image, the more violent the hatred. Or, if his own arrogance is repressed, he may blindly admire persons who are openly convinced of their importance and show it by arrogant behavior. He loves in them his own image and inevitably runs into severe disappointment when he becomes aware, as he must at some time or other, that the gods he so admires are interested only in themselves, and as far as he is concerned care only for the incense he burns at their altars.

Probably the worst drawback is the ensuing alienation from the self. We cannot suppress or eliminate essential parts of ourselves without becoming estranged from ourselves. It is one of those changes gradually produced by neurotic processes that despite their fundamental nature come about unobserved. The person simply becomes oblivious to what he really feels, likes, rejects, believes—in short, to what he really is. Without knowing it he may live the life of his image. Tommy in J. M. Barrie's *Tommy and Grizel* illuminates this process better than any clinical description. Of course it is not possible to behave so without being inextricably caught in a spider's web of unconscious pretense and rationalization, which makes for precarious living. The person loses interest in life because it is not he who lives it; he cannot make decisions because he does not know what he really wants; if difficulties mount, he may be pervaded by a sense of unreality—an accentuated expression of his permanent condition of being unreal to himself. To understand such a state we must realize that a veil of unreality shrouding the inner world is bound to be extended to the outer. A patient recently epitomized the whole situation by saying: "If it were not for reality, I would be quite all right."

Finally, although the idealized image is created to remove the basic conflict and in a limited way succeeds in doing so, it generates at the same time a new rift in the personality almost more dangerous than the original one. Roughly speaking, a person builds up an idealized image of himself because he cannot tolerate himself as he actually is. The image apparently counteracts this calamity; but having placed himself on a pedestal, he can tolerate his real self still less and starts to rage against it, to despise himself and to chafe under the yoke of his own unattainable demands upon himself. He wavers then between self-adoration and self-contempt, between his idealized image and his despised image, with no solid middle ground to fall back on.

Thus a new conflict is created between compulsive, contradictory strivings on the one hand and a kind of internal dictatorship imposed by the inner disturbance. And he reacts to this inner dictatorship just as a person might react to a comparable political dictatorship: he may identify himself with it, that is, feel that he is as wonderful and ideal as the dictator tells him he is; or he may stand on tiptoe to try to measure up to its demands; or he may rebel against the coercion and refuse to recognize the imposed obligations. If he reacts in the first way, we get the impression of a "narcissistic" individual, inaccessible to criticism; the existing rift, then, is not consciously felt as such. In the second instance we have the perfectionistic person, Freud's superego type. In the

third, the person appears not to be accountable to anyone or anything; he tends to become erratic, irresponsi-
ble, and negativistic. I speak advisedly of impressions
and appearances, because whatever is his reaction, he
continues to be fundamentally restive. Even a rebellious
type who ordinarily believes he is "free" labors under
the enforced standards he is trying to overthrow; though
the fact that he is still in the clutches of his idealized
image may show only in his swinging those standards
as a whip over others.[6] Sometimes a person goes through
periods of alternating between one extreme and another. He may, for instance, try for a time to be superhumanly "good" and, getting no comfort from that,
swing to the opposite pole of rebelling violently against
such standards. Or he may switch from an apparently
unreserved self-adoration to perfectionism. More often
we find a combination of these variant attitudes. All of
which points to the fact—understandable in the light
of our theory—that none of the attempts are satisfactory;
that they all are doomed to failure; that we must regard
them as desperate efforts to get out of an intolerable
situation; that as in any other intolerable situation the
most dissimilar means are tried—if one fails, another is
resorted to.

All these consequences combine to build a mighty
barrier against true development. The person cannot
learn from his mistakes because he does not see them.
In spite of his assertions to the contrary he is actually
bound to lose interest in his own growth. What he has
in mind when he speaks of growth is an unconscious

[6] *Cf.* Chapter 12, Sadistic Trends.

idea of creating a more perfect idealized image, one that will be without drawbacks.

The task of therapy, therefore, is to make the patient aware of his idealized image in all its detail, to assist him in gradually understanding all its functions and subjective values, and to show him the suffering that it inevitably entails. He will then start to wonder whether the price is not too high. But he can relinquish the image only when the needs that have created it are considerably diminished.

CHAPTER SEVEN

Externalization

WE HAVE seen how all the pretenses to which a neurotic resorts in order to bridge the gap between his real self and his idealized image serve in the end only to widen it. But because the image is of such tremendous subjective value he must continue unremittingly to try to come to terms with it. The ways in which he goes about this are manifold. Many of them will be discussed in the next chapter. Here we shall confine ourselves to examining one less well known than the rest, whose influence on the structure of neurosis is especially incisive.

When I call this attempt *externalization* I am defining the tendency to experience internal processes as if they occurred outside oneself and, as a rule, to hold these external factors responsible for one's difficulties. It has in common with idealization the purpose of getting away from the real self. But while the process of retouching and recreating the actual personality remains, as it were, within the precincts of self, externalization means abandoning the territory of self altogether. To put it simply, a person can take refuge from his basic conflict in his idealized image; but when discrepancies between the actual self and the idealized one reach a point where tensions become unbearable, he can no longer resort to anything within himself. The only thing left then is to run away from himself entirely and see everything as if it lay outside.

Some of the phenomena that occur here are covered by the term projection, meaning the objectifying of personal difficulties.[1] As commonly applied, projection means the shifting of blame and responsibility to someone else for subjectively rejected trends or qualities, such as suspecting others of one's own tendencies toward betrayal, ambition, domination, self-righteousness, meekness, and so on. In this sense the term is perfectly acceptable. Externalization, however, is a more comprehensive phenomenon; the shifting of responsibility is only a part of it. Not only one's faults are experienced in others but to a greater or less degree all feelings. A person who tends to externalize may be profoundly disturbed by the oppression of small countries, while unaware of how much he himself feels oppressed. He may not feel his own despair but will emotionally experience it in others. What is particularly important in this connection, he is unaware of his own attitudes toward himself; he will, for example, feel that someone else is angry with him when he actually is angry with himself. Or he will be conscious of anger at others that in reality he directs at himself. Further, he will ascribe not only his disturbances but also his good moods or achievements to external factors. While his failures will be seen as the decree of fate, his successes will be laid to fortuitous circumstances, his high spirits to the weather, and so on.

When a person feels that his life for good or ill is

[1] This definition was suggested by Edward A. Strecker and Kenneth E. Appel, *Discovering Ourselves*, Macmillan, 1943.

determined by others, it is only logical that he should be preoccupied with changing them, reforming them, punishing them, protecting himself from their interference, or impressing them. In this way externalization makes for dependence upon others—a dependence, however, quite different from that created by a neurotic need for affection. It also makes for overdependence upon external circumstances. Whether the person lives in the city or the suburbs, whether he keeps this or that diet, goes to bed early or late, serves on this or that committee, assumes undue importance. He thus acquires the characteristics that Jung calls extraversion. But while Jung regards extraversion as a one-sided development of constitutionally given trends, I see it as the result of trying to remove unsolved conflicts by externalization.

Another inevitable product of externalization is a gnawing sense of emptiness and shallowness. Again this feeling is not properly allocated. Instead of feeling the emotional emptiness as such, the person experiences it as emptiness in his stomach and tries to do away with it by compulsive eating. Or he may fear that his lack of bodily weight could cause him to be tossed about like a feather—any storm, he feels, might carry him away. He may even say that he would be nothing but an empty shell if everything were analyzed. The more thoroughgoing the externalization, the more the neurotic becomes wraithlike and apt merely to drift.

So much for the implications of this process. Let us see now how it specifically helps allay tension between the self and the idealized image. For no matter how a person may regard himself consciously, the disparity between the two will take an unconscious toll; and the more he has succeeded in identifying himself with the image, the more deeply unconscious will be the reaction. Most commonly it is expressed in self-contempt, rage against the self, and a feeling of coercion, all of which are not only extremely painful but in various ways incapacitate a person for living.

Externalization of self-contempt may take the form either of despising others or of feeling that it is others who look down upon oneself. Both forms are usually present; which is the more prominent, or at least the more conscious, depends on the whole setup of the neurotic character structure. The more aggressive a person is, the more right and superior he feels, the more readily will he despise others, and the less likely would it be to enter his mind that others could look down on him. Conversely, the more compliant he is, the more will his self-recriminations for his failure to measure up to his idealized image tend to make him feel that others have no use for him. The effect of the latter is particularly damaging. It makes a person shy, stilted, withdrawn. It makes him overgrateful—indeed abjectly grateful—for any affection or appreciation shown him. At the same time he cannot accept even sincere friendliness at its face value, but vaguely takes it for a kind of undeserved charity. He is rendered defenseless against arrogant persons because part of him agrees with them, and he feels that his being treated contemptuously is quite in order. Naturally such reactions breed resentment, which if repressed and piled up may gather explosive strength.

In spite of all this, experiencing self-contempt in an

externalized form has a distinct subjective value. To feel all his own scorn would smash whatever spurious self-assurance the neurotic may have and bring him to the verge of collapse. It is painful enough to be despised by others, but there is always hope of being able to change their attitude, or a prospect of paying them back in kind, or a mental reservation that they are unfair. When it is oneself one despises, all this is of no avail. There is no court of appeal. All the hopelessness the neurotic unconsciously feels in regard to himself would come into clear relief. He would start not only to despise his actual frailties but feel that he is altogether contemptible. Thus even his good qualities would be drawn into the abyss of his sense of unworthiness. In other words, he would feel himself to be his despised image; he would see it as an unalterable fact for which there was no help. This points to the advisability in therapeutic procedure of not touching upon self-contempt until the patient's hopelessness is diminished and the grip of the idealized image considerably loosened. Only then will the patient be able to face it and come to realize that his unworthiness is not an objective fact but a subjective feeling stemming from his merciless standards. In taking a more lenient attitude toward himself he will see that the condition is not unalterable, that the attributes he so objects to are not really despicable but are difficulties he can eventually overcome.

We shall not understand the neurotic's *rage at himself* or the dimensions it assumes unless we keep in mind how immeasurably important it is for him to maintain the illusion that he is his idealized image. The fact that he not only feels despair at his inability to measure up to it but is positively infuriated at himself is due to the sense of omnipotence that is an invariable attribute of the image. No matter how insurmountable the odds were against him in childhood, he, the omnipotent, should have been able to overcome them. Even if he realizes intellectually how great his neurotic entanglements are, he nonetheless feels an impotent rage at having been unable to dispel them. This rage reaches a climax when he is confronted with conflicting drives and realizes that even he is powerless to attain contradictory goals. This is one of the reasons why the sudden recognition of a conflict may throw him into a state of acute panic.

Rage at oneself is externalized in three main ways. Where giving vent to hostility is uninhibited, anger is easily thrust outward. It is turned then against others and appears either as irritability in general or as a specific irritation directed at the very faults in others that the person hates in himself. An illustration may make this clear. A patient complained of her husband's indecision. Since the indecision concerned a trivial matter, her vehemence was distinctly out of proportion. Knowing her own indecision, I suggested that she had revealed how mercilessly she condemned this in herself. Whereupon she suddenly felt an insane rage, with an impulse to tear herself to pieces. The fact that in her idealized image she was a tower of strength made it impossible for her to tolerate any weakness in herself. Characteristically enough, this reaction, in spite of its highly dramatic nature, was completely forgotten at the next interview. She had seen the externalization in a flash but was not yet ready to relinquish it.

The second way takes the form of an incessant conscious or unconscious fear or expectation that the faults which are intolerable to oneself will infuriate others. A person may be so convinced that certain behavior on his part will arouse profound hostility that he may be honestly bewildered if no hostile response is encountered. A patient, for instance, whose idealized image contained elements of wanting to be as good as the priest in Victor Hugo's *Les Misérables,* was greatly astonished to find that whenever she took a firm stand or even expressed anger, people liked her better than when she acted like a saint. As one would guess from this kind of idealized image, the patient's predominant trend was compliance. Issuing originally from her need for closeness to others, it was greatly reinforced by her expectation of hostile response. Increased compliance is in fact one of the major consequences of this form of externalization, and illustrates how neurotic trends continually augment each other in a vicious circle. Compulsive compliance is increased because the idealized image, containing in this configuration elements of saintliness, drives the person to greater self-effacement. The resulting hostile impulses then arouse rage against the self. And the externalization of the rage, leading to an increased fear of others, in turn reinforces compliance.

The third way of externalizing rage is to focus on bodily disorders. Rage against the self, when not experienced as such, apparently creates physical tensions of considerable severity, which may appear as intestinal maladies, headaches, fatigue, and so on. It is illuminating to see how all these symptoms disappear with the speed of lightning as soon as the rage itself is consciously felt. One may be in doubt whether to call these physical manifestations externalization or to regard them merely as physiological consequences of repressed rage. But one can hardly separate the manifestations from the use patients make of them. As a rule they are more than eager to ascribe their psychic troubles to their bodily ailments and these in turn to some external provocation. There is nothing psychically wrong with them, they are interested to prove; they just suffer from intestinal troubles due to wrong diet, or from fatigue due to overwork, or from rheumatism due to damp air, and so on and so on.

As to what the neurotic accomplishes by externalizing his rage, the same may be said here as in the case of self-contempt. One additional consideration should, however, be mentioned. The lengths to which such patients go will not be fully understood unless one is cognizant of the real danger attached to these self-destructive impulses. The patient cited in the first example had only a momentary impulse to tear herself to pieces, but psychotics may really carry it through and mutilate themselves.[2] It is probable that many more suicides would occur if it were not for externalization. It is understandable that Freud, being aware of the power of self-destructive impulses, should have postu-

[2] Many illustrations of this will be found in Karl Menninger, *Man against Himself*, Harcourt, Brace, 1938. Menninger, however, approaches the subject from an entirely different angle, in that—following Freud—he assumes a self-destructive instinct.

lated a self-destructive instinct (death instinct)—though by this concept he barred the way to a real understanding, and so to an effective therapy.

The intensity of the *feeling of inner coercion* depends on the extent to which the personality is cramped by the authoritative control of the idealized image. It would be hard to overestimate this pressure. It is worse than any external coercion because the latter permits inner freedom to be retained. Patients are for the most part unaware of the feeling, but one can gauge its power by their relief when it is removed and a measure of inner freedom acquired. The coercion may be externalized on the one hand by imposing pressure upon others. This can have the same outward effect as a neurotic craving for domination, but though both may be present they differ in that coercion which represents an externalization of inner pressure is not primarily a demand for personal obedience. It consists chiefly in imposing the same standards upon others as those under which the person himself chafes—and with the same disregard for their happiness. Puritan psychology is a well-known illustration of this process.

Equally important is the externalization of this inner compulsion in the form of hypersensitivity to anything in the outside world that even faintly resembles duress. As every observant person knows, such hypersensitivity is common. Not all of it stems from self-imposed coercion. Usually there is an element of experiencing one's own power drive in others and resenting it. In detached personalities we think primarily of the compulsive insistence upon independence that would necessarily make them sensitive to any outside pressure. Externalization of an unconscious self-imposed constraint is a source that is more hidden and more often neglected in analysis. This is particularly regrettable since it often constitutes an influential undercurrent in the relationship between patient and analyst. The patient is likely to keep on invalidating every suggestion made by the analyst even after the more obvious sources of his sensitivity on this score have been analyzed. The subversive battle set afoot in this event is all the more severe because the analyst actually does want to bring about changes in the patient. His honest assertion that he merely wants to help the patient retrieve himself and the inner springs of his life is of little avail. Might he, the patient, not succumb to some inadvertently exerted influence? The fact is that since he does not know what he "really" is, he cannot possibly be selective in what he accepts or rejects, and no amount of care on the analyst's part to refrain from imposing any personally held belief will make any difference. And since he also does not know that he labors under an inner coercion which has set him in a certain pattern, he can only rebel indiscriminately against every external intent to change him. Needless to say, this futile battle appears not only in the analytical situation but is bound to occur in greater or less degree in any close relationship. It is the analysis of this inner process that will finally lay the ghost.

To complicate matters, the more a person tends to comply with the exacting demands of his idealized image the more will he externalize such compliance. He will be eager to measure up to what the analyst—or anybody else, for that matter—expects of him or what he believes they expect of him. He may appear amenable or even gullible but at the same time he will pile up secret resentment against this "coercion." The result may be that he will eventually come to see everyone in a dominating role and be universally resentful.

What, then, does a person gain by externalizing his inner constraint? As long as he believes it comes from outside he can rebel against it, even if only by way of mental reservation. Similarly, a restriction externally imposed can be avoided; an illusion of freedom can be maintained. But more significant is the factor cited above: to admit the inner coercion would mean to admit that he is not his idealized image, with all the consequences that entails.

It is an interesting question whether and to what extent the strain of this inner compulsion, too, is expressed in physical symptoms. My own impression is that it is a contributing factor in asthma, high blood pressure, and constipation, but my experience here is limited.

It remains for us to discuss the externalization of the various features that stand in contrast to one's idealized image. This on the whole is effected by simple projection—that is, by experiencing them in others or by holding others responsible for them. The two processes do not necessarily go together. In the following examples we may have to repeat certain things we have already said in this connection, as well as others that are commonly known, but the illustrations will help us to arrive at a deeper understanding of the meaning of projection.

An alcoholic patient, A, complained of the inconsid-

erateness of his mistress. As far as I could see, the complaint was not warranted, or at any rate not nearly
to the extent that A implied. He himself suffered from
a conflict, quite obvious to an outsider, of being compliant, good-natured, and generous on the one hand
and domineering, demanding, and arrogant on the
other. Here, then, was a projection of aggressive trends.
But what made the projection necessary? In his idealized image, aggressive tendencies were merely a natural
ingredient of a forceful personality. The most prominent feature, however, was goodness—there had not
been anyone so good as he since St. Francis, and never
had there been such an ideal friend. Was the projection, then, a sop to his idealized image? Certainly! But
it also permitted him to live out his aggressive trends
without becoming aware of them and so being confronted with his conflicts. Here was a person caught in
an unsolvable dilemma. He could not relinquish his
aggressive trends because they were of a compulsive
nature. Neither could he abandon his idealized image,
for it was what held him together. The projection was
a way out of the dilemma. It thus represented an *unconscious duplicity:* it enabled him to assert all his arrogant demands and to be at the same time the ideal
friend.

The patient also suspected the woman of infidelity.
There was no evidence for this whatsoever—she was
devoted to him in a rather maternal way. The fact was
that he himself was given to transitory affairs which
he kept secret. One might think here of a retaliatory
fear growing out of his judging others by himself. Certainly a need to justify himself was involved. Considera-

tion of a possible projection of homosexual tendencies did not help to clarify the situation. The clue lay in his peculiar attitude toward his own unfaithfulness. His affairs were not forgotten, but in retrospect they did not register. They were no longer a live experience. The alleged unfaithfulness of the woman, on the other hand, was quite vivid. Here, then, was an externalization of experience. Its function was the same as that of the previous example: it allowed him to maintain the idealized image and also do as he pleased.

Power politics, as played among political and professional groups, may serve as another instance. Frequently such maneuvering is motivated by a conscious intention to weaken a rival and fortify one's own position. But it may also spring from an unconscious dilemma similar to the one presented above. In that case it would be an expression of unconscious duplicity. It would permit one all the intrigue and manipulation involved in this kind of attack without blemishing the idealized image, while at the same time affording an excellent way of pouring all one's anger and contempt for oneself upon another person—better still, upon one whom it is desirable to defeat in the first place.

I shall conclude by pointing out a common way in which responsibility may be shifted to others without investing them with one's own difficulties. Many patients, as soon as they are made aware of certain of their problems, jump immediately to their childhood and pin all their explanations on that. They are sensitive to coercion, they say, because they had a domineering mother. They are easily humiliated because humiliations were suffered in childhood; they are vindictive because of their early injuries; they are withdrawn because nobody understood them when they were young; they are sexually inhibited because of their puritanical upbringing, and so on and so on. I do not refer here to interviews in which both analyst and patient are seriously engaged in understanding early influences but rather to an overeagerness to explore childhood which leads to nothing but endless repetition and is accompanied by an equally great lack of interest in exploring the forces operating in the patient at present.

Inasmuch as this attitude is supported by Freud's overemphasis on genesis, let us carefully examine how much of it is based on truth and how much on fallacy. It is true that the patient's neurotic development started in childhood and that all the data he can provide is relevant to an understanding of the specific kind of development that has taken place. It is true also that he is not responsible for his neurosis. The impact of circumstances was such that he could not help developing as he did. For reasons that will be discussed presently, the analyst must make this point very clear.

The fallacy lies in the patient's lack of interest in all the forces that have been built up in him on the basis of his childhood. These, however, are the forces that are operating in him now and that lie behind the present difficulties. His having seen so much hypocrisy around him as a child may have played a part, for instance, in making him cynical. But if he relates his cynicism to his early experience alone, he ignores his current need to be cynical—a need that springs from his being divided between divergent ideals and so having to throw all values overboard in an attempt to solve that conflict. Moreover, he tends to assume responsibility where he cannot, and to refuse to assume it where he should. He keeps referring to early experiences in order to reassure himself that he really cannot help having certain failings, and at the same time feels that he should have come out of his early calamities unscathed—a white lily emerging unsullied from a bog. For this his idealized image is partly to blame, since it will not permit him to accept himself with flaws or conflicts past or present. But more important, his harping on childhood is a particular kind of evasion of self which still allows him to maintain an illusion of eagerness for self-scrutiny. Because he externalizes them he does not experience the forces operating within him; and he cannot conceive of himself as an active instrument in his own life. Having ceased to be the propellant, he thinks of himself as a ball that once pushed downhill must keep on rolling, or as a guinea pig, once conditioned forever determined.

The one-sided emphasis a patient may put on childhood is so definite an expression of his externalizing tendencies that whenever I meet this attitude I expect to find a person who is thoroughly alienated from himself and who continues to be driven centrifugally away from himself. And I have not yet been mistaken in this anticipation.

The tendency to externalize operates in dreams as well. If the analyst appears in the patient's dreams as a jailer, if the husband slams the doors through which the dreamer wants to pass, if accidents occur or obstacles interfere with reaching a much desired destination, these dreams constitute an attempt to deny the inner conflict and to ascribe it to some external factor.

A patient with a general tendency to externalize

offers peculiar difficulties in analysis. He comes to it as he would go to a dentist, expecting the analyst to perform a job that does not really concern him. He is interested in the neurosis of his wife, friend, brother, but not in his own. He talks about the difficult circumstances under which he lives and is reluctant to examine his share in them. If his wife were not so neurotic or his work so upsetting, he would be quite all right. For a considerable period he has no realization whatever that any emotional forces could possibly be operating within himself; he is afraid of ghosts, burglars, thunderstorms, of vindictive persons around him, of the political situation, but never of himself. He is at best interested in his problems for the intellectual or artistic pleasure they afford him. But as long as he is, so to speak, psychically nonexistent, he cannot possibly apply any insight he may gain to his actual living, and therefore in spite of his greater knowledge about himself can change very little.

Externalization is thus essentially an active process of self-elimination. The reason for its being feasible at all lies in the estrangement from the self that is inherent in the neurotic process anyhow. With the self eliminated, it is only natural that the inner conflicts, too, should be removed from awareness. But by making the person more reproachful, vindictive, and fearful in respect to others, externalization replaces the inner conflicts with external ones. More specifically, it greatly aggravates the conflict that originally set in motion the whole neurotic process: the conflict between the individual and the outer world.

CHAPTER EIGHT

Auxiliary Approaches to Artificial Harmony

IT IS A commonplace that one lie usually leads to another, the second takes a third to bolster it, and so on till one is caught in a tangled web. Something of the sort is bound to happen in any situation in the life of an individual or group where a determination to go to the root of the matter is lacking. The patchwork may be of some help, but it will generate new problems which in turn require a new makeshift. So it is with neurotic attempts to solve the basic conflict; and here, as elsewhere, nothing is of any real avail but a radical change in the conditions out of which the original difficulty arose. What the neurotic does instead—and cannot help doing—is to pile one pseudo solution upon another. He may try, as we have seen, to make one face of the conflict predominate. He remains as torn as ever. He may resort to the drastic measure of detaching himself from others entirely; but though the conflict is set out of operation his whole life is put on a precarious basis. He creates an idealized self in which he appears triumphant and unified, but at the same time creates a new rift. He tries to do away with that rift by eliminating his inner self from the field of combat, only to find himself in an even more intolerable predicament.

So unstable an equilibrium requires still further measures to support it. He turns then to any one of a number of unconscious devices, which may be classified as blind spots, compartmentalizing, rationalizing, excessive self-control, arbitrary rightness, elusiveness, and cynicism. We shall not attempt to discuss these phenomena *per se*—that would be too intensive a task—but will show only how they are employed in connection with conflicts.

The discrepancy between a neurotic's actual behavior and his idealized picture of himself can be so blatant that one wonders how he himself can help seeing it. But far from doing so, he is able to remain unaware of a contradiction that stares him in the face. This *blind spot* in view of the most obvious contradictions was one of the first things that drew my attention to the existence and relevance of the conflicts I have described. A patient, for example, who had all the characteristics of the compliant type and thought of himself as Christlike, told me quite casually that at staff meetings he would often shoot one colleague after another with a little flick of his thumb. True enough, the destructive craving that prompted these figurative killings was at that time unconscious; but the point here is that the shooting, which he dubbed "play," did not in the least disturb his Christlike image.

Another patient, a scientist who believed himself seriously devoted to his work and considered himself an innovator in his field, was guided in his choice of what he should publish by purely opportunistic motives, presenting only papers that he felt would bring him the most acclaim. There was no attempt at camouflage—merely the same blissful obliviousness to the con-

tradition involved. Similarly, a man who in his idealized image was goodness and straightforwardness itself
thought nothing of taking money from one girl to
spend it on another.

It is obvious that in each of these cases the function
of the blindness was to keep underlying conflicts from
awareness. What is amazing is the extent to which this
was possible, the more so since the patients in question
were not only intelligent but psychologically informed.
To say that we all tend to turn our backs on what we
do not care to see is surely insufficient explanation. We
should have to add that the degree to which we blot
out things depends on how great our interest is in doing
so. All in all, such artificial blindness demonstrates in
a quite simple fashion how great is our aversion to
recognizing conflicts. But the real problem here is how
we can manage to overlook contradictions as conspicuous as those just cited. The fact is that there are special
conditions without which it would indeed be impossible. One of them is an inordinate numbness to our
own emotional experience. The other, already pointed
out by Strecker,[1] is the phenomenon of living in *compartments*. Strecker, who also offers illustrations of the
blind spots, speaks of logic-tight compartments and
segregation. There is a section for friends and one for
enemies, one for the family and one for outsiders, one
for professional and one for personal life, one for social
equals and one for inferiors. Hence what happens in
one compartment does not appear to the neurotic to
contradict what happens in another. It is possible for
a person to live that way only when, by reason of his

[1] Strecker, *op. cit.*

conflicts, he has lost his sense of unity. Compartmentalizing is thus as much a result of being divided by one's
conflicts as a defense against recognizing them. The
process is not unlike that described in the case of one
kind of idealized image: contradictions remain, but the
conflicts are spirited away. It is hard to say whether this
type of idealized image is responsible for the compartmentalization or the other way around. It seems likely,
however, that the fact of living in compartments is the
more fundamental and that it would account for the
kind of image created.

To appreciate this phenomenon, cultural factors
must be taken into consideration. Man has become to
so great a degree merely a cog in an intricate social system that alienation from the self is almost universal,
and human values themselves have declined. As a result
of innumerable outstanding contradictions in our civilization a general numbness of moral perception has developed. Moral standards are so casually regarded that
no one is surprised, for instance, to see a person a pious
Christian or a devoted father one day, conducting himself like a gangster the next.[2] There are too few wholehearted and integrated persons around us to offer contrast to our own scatteredness. In the analytical situation Freud's discarding of moral values—a consequence
of his viewing psychology as a natural science—has contributed toward making the analyst just as blind as
the patient to contradictions of this sort. The analyst
thinks it "unscientific" to have moral values of his own
or to take any interest in those of the patient. As a matter of fact, the acceptance of contradictions appears in

[2] Lin Yutang, *Between Tears and Laughter,* John Day, 1943.

many theoretical formulations not necessarily confined to the moral sphere.

Rationalization may be defined as self-deception by reasoning. The common idea that it is primarily used to justify oneself or to bring one's motives and actions into accord with accepted ideologies is only valid up to a point; the implication there would be that persons living in the same civilization all rationalize along the same lines, whereas actually there is a wide range of individual difference in what is rationalized as well as in the methods employed. That this should be so is only natural if we view rationalization as one way of supporting neurotic attempts to create artificial harmony. In each of the planks of the defensive scaffolding built around the basic conflict, the process can be seen at work. The predominant attitude is strengthened by reasoning—factors that would bring the conflict into sight are either minimized or so remodeled as to fit in with it. How this self-deceptive reasoning aids the streamlining of the personality shows up when one contrasts the compliant type with the aggressive. The former ascribes his desire to be helpful to his sympathetic feelings, even though strong tendencies to dominate are present; and if these are too conspicuous he rationalizes them as solicitousness. The latter, when he is helpful, firmly denies any feeling of sympathy and lays his action entirely to expediency. The idealized image always requires a good deal of rationalization for its support: discrepancies between the actual self and the image must be reasoned out of existence. In externalizing, it is brought to bear to prove the relevance of outside circumstances or to show that the traits unacceptable to the individual himself are merely a "natural" reaction to the behavior of others.

The tendency toward *excessive self-control* can be so strong that I at one time counted it among the original neurotic trends.[3] Its function is to serve as a dam against being flooded by contradictory emotions. Though in the beginning it is often an act of conscious will power, in time it usually becomes more or less automatic. Persons who exert such control will not allow themselves to be carried away, whether by enthusiasm, sexual excitement, self-pity, or rage. In analysis they have the greatest difficulty in associating freely; they will not permit alcohol to lift their spirits and frequently prefer to endure pain rather than undergo anesthesia. In short, they seek to check all spontaneity. This trait is most strongly developed in individuals whose conflicts are fairly out in the open, those who have not taken either of the steps that ordinarily help to submerge the conflicts; clear predominance has not been given to one of the conflicting sets of attitudes, nor has sufficient detachment been developed to put the conflicts out of operation. Such persons are held together merely by their idealized image; and apparently its binding power is insufficient when unaided by one or the other of the primary attempts at establishing inner unity. The image is particularly inadequate when it takes the form of a composite of contradictory elements. The exertion of will power then, consciously or unconsciously, is needed to keep the conflicting impulses under control. Since the most disruptive impulses are those of violence

[3] Karen Horney, *Self-Analysis, op. cit.*

prompted by rage, the greatest degree of energy is directed toward the control of rage. Here a vicious circle is set in motion; the rage, by reason of being suppressed, attains explosive strength, which in turn requires still more self-control to choke it. If the patient's excessive control is brought to his attention he will defend it by pointing to the virtue and necessity of self-control for any civilized individual. What he overlooks is the compulsive nature of his control. He cannot help exerting it in the most rigid way and is seized by panic if for any reason it fails to function. The panic may appear as a fear of insanity, which clearly indicates that the function of the control is to ward off the danger of being split apart.

Arbitrary rightness has the twofold function of eliminating doubt from within and influence from without. Doubt and indecision are invariable concomitants of unresolved conflicts and can reach an intensity powerful enough to paralyze all action. In such a state a person is naturally susceptible to influence. When we have genuine convictions we will not be readily swayed; but if all our lives we stand at a crossroad, undecided whether to go in this direction or that, outside agencies can easily be the determining factor, if only temporarily. Moreover, indecision applies not only to possible courses of action but also includes doubts about oneself, one's rights, one's worth.

All these uncertainties detract from our ability to cope with life. Apparently, however, they are not equally intolerable to everyone. The more a person sees life as a merciless battle, the more will he regard doubt as a dangerous weakness. The more isolated he is and insistent upon independence, the more will susceptibility to foreign influence be a source of irritation. All my observation points to the fact that a combination of predominant aggressive trends and detachment is the most fertile soil for the development of rigid rightness; and the nearer to the surface the aggression, the more militant the rightness. It constitutes an attempt to settle conflicts once and for all by declaring arbitrarily and dogmatically that one is invariably right. In a system so governed by rationality, emotions are traitors from within and must be checked by unswerving control. Peace may be attained but it is the peace of the grave. As would be expected, such persons loathe the idea of analysis because it threatens to disarrange the tidy picture.

Almost polar to rigid rightness, but likewise an effective defense against the recognition of conflicts, is *elusiveness*. Patients inclined toward this kind of defense often resemble those characters in fairy tales who when pursued turn into fish; if not safe in this guise, they turn into deer; if the hunter catches up with them they fly away as birds. You can never pin them down to any statement; they deny having said it or assure you they did not mean it that way. They have a bewildering capacity to becloud issues. It is often impossible for them to give a concrete report of any incident; should they try to do so the listener is uncertain in the end just what really did happen.

The same confusion reigns in their lives. They are vicious one moment, sympathetic the next; at times overconsiderate, ruthlessly inconsiderate at others; domineering in some respects, self-effacing in others. They reach out for a dominating partner, only to change to a "doormat," then back to the former variety. After treating someone badly, they will be overcome by remorse, attempt to make amends, then feel like a "sucker" and turn to being abusive all over again. Nothing is quite real to them.

The analyst may well find himself confused, and, discouraged, feel there is no substance to work with. There he is mistaken. These are simply patients who have not succeeded in adopting the customary unifying procedures: they have not only failed to repress parts of their conflict, but they have established no definite idealized image. In a way they may be said to demonstrate the value of these attempts. For no matter how troublesome the consequences, persons who have so proceeded are better organized and not nearly so lost as the elusive type. On the other hand, the analyst would be equally mistaken were he to count on an easy job by virtue of the fact that the conflicts are visible and need not therefore be dragged out of hiding. Nevertheless he will find himself up against the patient's aversion to any transparency, and this will tend to defeat him unless he himself understands that this is the patient's way of warding off any real insight.

A final defense against the recognition of conflicts is *cynicism,* the denying and deriding of moral values. A deep-seated uncertainty in respect to moral values is bound to be present in every neurosis, no matter how dogmatically the person adheres to the particular aspects of his standards that are acceptable to him. While the genesis of cynicism varies, its function invariably is to deny the existence of moral values, thereby relieving the neurotic of the necessity of making clear to himself what it is he actually believes in.

Cynicism can be conscious, and then become a principle in the Machiavellian tradition and be so defended. All that counts is appearance. You can do as you please as long as you don't get caught. Everyone is a hypocrite who isn't fundamentally stupid. This kind of patient may be as sensitive to the analyst's using the term moral, regardless of the context, as those of Freud's time were to the mention of sex. But cynicism may also remain unconscious and be concealed by lip service to prevalent ideologies. Unaware though he may be of the hold his cynicism has upon him, the way he lives and the way he talks about his life will reveal that he acts upon its principles. Or he may involve himself unwittingly in contradictions, like the patient who was sure he believed in honesty and decency yet was envious of anyone who indulged in crooked maneuvers and resented the fact that he himself never "got away" with that kind of thing. In therapy it is important to bring the patient's cynicism to full awareness at the proper time and help him to understand it. It may also be necessary to explain why it is desirable for him to establish his own set of moral values.

The foregoing, then, are the defenses built around the nucleus of the basic conflict. For simplicity I shall refer to the whole system of defense as the protective structure. A combination of defenses is developed in every neurosis; often all of them are present, though in varying degrees of activity.

PART II

*Consequences of
Unresolved Conflicts*

CHAPTER NINE

Fears

IN SEARCHING for the deeper meaning of any neurotic problem we can easily lose our bearings in a maze of intricacies. This is not unnatural, since we cannot hope to understand neurosis without facing its complexity. It is helpful, though, to stand aside from time to time in order to regain our perspective.

We have followed the development of the protective structure step by step. We have seen how one defense after another is built up until a comparatively static organization is established. And the element that impresses us most deeply in all this is the infinite labor that has gone into the process, a labor so tremendous that we are led again to wonder what it is that drives a person along so arduous a path and one so fraught with cost to himself. We ask ourselves what are the forces that make the structure so rigid and so difficult to change. Is the motive power of the whole process simply the fear of the disruptive potency of the basic conflict? An analogy may clear a way to the answer. Like any analogy it is not a precise parallel and so can only be applied in the broadest terms. Let us assume that a man with a shady past has found his way into a community by false pretense. He will, of course, live in dread of his former state's being disclosed. In the course of time his situation advances; he makes friends, secures a job, founds a family. Cherishing his new position, he is beset with a new fear, the fear of losing these goods. His pride in his respectability alienates him from his unsavory past. He gives large sums to charity and even to his old associates in order to wipe out his old life. Meanwhile the changes that have been taking place in his personality proceed to involve him in new conflicts, with the result that in the end his having commenced his present life on false premises becomes merely an undercurrent in his disturbance.

So in the organization the neurotic has established, the basic conflict remains but is transmuted. Tempered in some respects, it is enhanced in others. Due, however, to the vicious circle inherent in the process, the ensuing conflicts become more urgent. What sharpens them most is the fact that every fresh defensive position further impairs his relations with himself and others— the soil, as we have seen, out of which conflicts grow. Moreover, as new elements, however wrapped in illusion—love or success, an achieved detachment or an established image—come to play an important part in his life, a fear of a different order is generated, the fear that something may jeopardize these treasures. And all the while, his increased alienation from himself deprives him more and more of the capacity to work on himself and so get rid of his difficulties. Inertia sets in, taking the place of a directed growth.

The protective structure, for all its rigidity, is highly brittle and itself gives rise to new fears. One of these is a fear that its *equilibrium will be disturbed*. While the structure lends a sense of balance, it is a balance that is easily upset. The person himself is not consciously aware of this threat, but he cannot help feeling it in a variety of ways. Experience has taught him that he can be thrown out of gear for no apparent reason, that he becomes infuriated, elated, depressed, fatigued, inhibited when he least anticipates or desires it. The sum total of such experiences gives him a feeling of uncertainty, a feeling that he cannot rely on himself. It is as if he were skating on thin ice. His imbalance may also be expressed in gait or posture, or in lack of skill in anything requiring physical balance.

The most concrete expression of this fear is a fear of insanity. When that is present in a marked degree it can be the paramount symptom that drives a person to seek psychiatric help. In such instances the fear is also determined by repressed impulses to do all sorts of "crazy" things, mostly of a destructive nature, without feeling responsible for them. The fear of insanity, however, is not to be construed as an indication that the person may actually go insane. Usually it is transitory and emerges only under conditions of acute distress. Its most poignant provocations are a sudden threat to the idealized image, or a mounting tension—most commonly due to unconscious rage—that puts excessive self-control in jeopardy. A woman, for example, who believed herself to be both even-tempered and courageous had an onset of panic when, in a difficult situation, she was struck with a feeling of helplessness, apprehension, and violent anger. Her idealized image, which had held her together as with a band of steel, suddenly burst and left her with a fear of going to pieces. We have already spoken of the panic that may seize a detached person when he is pulled from his shelter and brought into close proximity to others—when, for instance, he has to join the army or live with relatives. This terror, too, may be expressed as a fear of insanity; and in this instance psychotic episodes may actually occur. In analysis a like fear will emerge when a patient who has gone to great lengths to create an artificial harmony suddenly recognizes that he is divided.

That fear of insanity is most frequently precipitated by unconscious rage is demonstrated in analysis when, this fear having subsided, its residues take the form of an apprehension that one may insult, beat, or even kill people under conditions where self-control is impossible. The commission of an act of violence in sleep or under the influence of drink, anesthesia, or sexual excitement will then be feared. The rage itself may be conscious or it may appear in consciousness as an obsessive impulse toward violence, unconnected with any affect. On the other hand it may be entirely unconscious; in that case all the person feels are sudden spells of vague panic, accompanied perhaps by perspiration, dizziness, or a fear of fainting—signifying an underlying fear that the violent impulses might get out of control. Where the unconscious rage is externalized, the person may have a terror of thunderstorms, ghosts, burglars, snakes, and so on—that is, of any potentially destructive force outside himself.

But after all, fear of insanity is comparatively rare. It is simply the most conspicuous expression of the fear of losing equilibrium. Ordinarily that fear operates in more hidden ways. It appears then in vague, indefinite forms and can be precipitated by any change in life's routine. Persons subject to it may feel profoundly disturbed at the prospect of making a journey or of moving or changing jobs or employing a new maid or whatever. Wherever possible they try to avoid such changes. Its threat to stability may be a factor in deterring patients from being analyzed, particularly if they have found a way of living that permits them to function fairly well. When they discuss the advisability of analysis they will be concerned about questions that at first glance seem reasonable enough: Will analysis uproot their marriage? Will it temporarily incapacitate them for work? Will it make them irritable? Will it interfere with their religion? As we shall see, such questions are in part determined by the patient's hopelessness; he does not think it worth while to take any risks. But there is also a real apprehension behind his concern: he needs to be reassured that analysis will not upset his equilibrium. In such cases we can safely assume that the equilibrium is particularly shaky and that the analysis will be a difficult one.

Can the analyst give the patient the assurance he wants? No, he cannot. Every analysis is bound to create temporary upsets. What the analyst can do, however, is to go to the root of such questions, to explain to the patient what he really is afraid of, and tell him that while analysis will upset his present balance it will give him an opportunity to attain an equilibrium more solidly grounded.

Another fear born of the protective structure is a *fear of exposure*. Its source lies in the many pretenses that go into the development and maintenance of the structure itself. These will be described in connection with the impairment of moral integrity brought about by unresolved conflicts. For our present purpose we need only point out that a neurotic person wants to appear, both to himself and others, different from what he really is—more harmonious, more rational, more generous or powerful or ruthless. It would be hard to say whether he is more afraid of being exposed to himself or to others. Consciously, it is others he is most concerned about, and the more he externalizes his fear the more anxious he is that others should not find him out. He may say in that case that what he thinks of himself does not matter; his own discovery of his failings he can take in his stride, if only others can be kept in the dark. This is not so, but it is the way he feels consciously and indicates the degree to which externalization is present.

Fear of being exposed may either appear as a nebulous feeling that one is a bluff or may be attached to some particular quality only remotely associated with what one is really bothered about. A person may be afraid that he is not as intelligent, as competent, as well educated, as attractive as he is believed to be, so shifting the fear to qualities that do not reflect on his character. Thus a patient recalled that in his early adolescence he was haunted by the fear that his being at the head of his class was due entirely to bluffing. Each time he changed schools he was sure that this time he would be found out, and the fear persisted even when again he captured the top rank. His feeling puzzled him, but he was unable to put his finger on the cause of it. He could not gain an insight into his problem because he was on the wrong track: his fear of exposure did not at all concern his intelligence but had merely been shifted to that sphere. In reality it concerned his unconscious pretense of being a good fellow who did not care about grades, whereas the fact was that he was obsessed by a destructive need to triumph over others. This illustration leads to a pertinent generalization. Fear of being a bluff is always related to some objective factor, but it is usually not the one the person himself thinks it is. Symptomatically, its outstanding expression is blushing or a fear of blushing. Since it is an unconscious pretense that the patient fears will be disclosed, the analyst will make a serious mistake if, noting the patient's fear of being found out, he searches for some experience that he thinks the latter is ashamed of and is hiding. But the patient may not be holding back anything of the sort. What happens then is that he becomes more and more fearful that there must be something particularly bad in him which he is unconsciously loath to reveal. Such a situation is conducive to self-condemnatory scrutiny but not to constructive work. He will perhaps go into further detail about sexual episodes or destructive impulses. But the fear of exposure will remain so long as the analyst fails to recognize that the patient is caught in a conflict and that he himself is working on only one aspect of it.

Fear of exposure can be provoked by any situation which—to the neurotic—means being put to a test. This would include starting a new job, making new friends, entering a new school, examinations, social gatherings, or any kind of performance that might make him conspicuous even if it is no more than taking part in a discussion. Frequently what is consciously conceived as a fear of failure actually has to do with exposure, and hence is not allayed by success. The person will merely feel that he "got by" this time, but what about the next? And if he should fail, he will only be the more convinced that he has always been a bluff and that this time he was caught. One consequence of such a feeling is shyness, particularly in any new situation. Another is wariness in the face of being liked or appreciated. The person will think, consciously or unconsciously: "They like me now, but if they really knew me they would feel otherwise." Naturally this fear plays a role in analysis, whose explicit purpose is to "find out."

Every new fear requires a new set of defenses. Those erected against fear of exposure fall into opposite categories and hinge on the whole character structure. On the one hand there is a tendency to avoid test situations of any kind; and if they cannot be avoided, to be reserved, self-controlled, and wear an impenetrable mask. On the other hand there is an unconscious attempt to become so perfect a bluff that exposure need not be feared. The latter attitude is not defensive alone: magnificent bluffing is also used by individuals of the aggressive type who live vicariously, as a means of impressing those whom they wish to exploit; any attempt to question them, then, will be met by a wily counterattack. I refer here to openly sadistic persons. We shall see later how this trait fits in with the entire structure.

We shall understand the fear of exposure when we have answered two questions: What is a person afraid to disclose? and, What is it that he fears in case he should be exposed? The first we have already answered. In order to answer the second we must deal with still another fear emanating from the protective structure, the fear of *disregard, humiliation,* and *ridicule.* While the ricketiness of the structure is responsible for the fear of a disturbed equilibrium, and the unconscious fraudulence involved breeds fear of exposure, the fear of humiliation comes from an injured self-esteem. We have touched on this matter in other connections. Both the creation of an idealized image and the process of externalization are attempts at repairing damaged self-respect, but as we have seen, both only injure it still further.

If we take a bird's-eye view of what happens to self-esteem in the course of a neurotic development, we come upon two pairs of seesaw processes. While the level of realistic self-esteem falls, up comes an unrealistic pride—pride in being so good, so aggressive, so unique, so omnipotent or omniscient. On the other seesaw we find a dwarfing of the neurotic's actual self counterweighted by the raising of others to the stature of giants. Through the eclipse of large areas of the self by repression and inhibition as well as by idealization and externalization, the individual loses sight of himself; he feels, if he does not actually become, like a shadow without weight or substance. And meanwhile his need of others and his fear of them make them not only more formidable to him but more necessary. Hence his center of gravity comes to rest more in others than in himself and he concedes to them prerogatives that are rightly his own. Its effect is to give their evaluation of himself undue importance, while his own self-evaluation loses significance. This lends to the opinion of others an overwhelming power.

The above sets of processes taken together account for the neurotic's extreme vulnerability to disregard, humiliation, and ridicule. And these processes are so much a part of every neurosis that hypersensitivity in this respect is most common. If we are cognizant of the manifold sources of the fear of disregard we can see that to remove or even diminish it is no simple task. It can recede only to the extent that the entire neurosis recedes.

In general, the consequence of this fear is to set the neurotic apart from others and make him hostile to them. But more important is its power to clip the wings of those afflicted with it to any strong degree. They do not dare to expect anything of others or to set high goals for themselves. They do not dare to approach people who seem superior to them in any way; they do not dare to express an opinion even though they may have a real contribution to make; they do not dare to exercise creative abilities even when they have them; they do not dare to make themselves attractive, to try to impress, to seek a better position, and so on and so on. When tempted to reach out in any of these directions the ghastly prospect of ridicule holds them back and they take refuge in reserve and dignity.

More imperceptible than the fears we have described is one that may be regarded as a condensation of all of them as well as of other fears that arise in a neurotic development. This is the fear of *changing anything in oneself*. Patients react to the idea of changing by adopting either of two extreme attitudes. They either leave the whole subject nebulous, feeling that a change will occur by some sort of miracle at some hazy future time, or they attempt to change too rapidly, with too little understanding. In the first instance they harbor a mental reservation that catching a glimpse of a problem or admitting a frailty should be enough; the idea that in order to fulfill themselves they must actually change their attitudes and drives comes as a shock to them and makes them uneasy. They cannot help seeing the validity of the proposition, but unconsciously they reject it all the same. The reverse position amounts to an unconscious pretense of changing. It is in part wishful thinking, growing out of the patient's intolerance of any imperfection in himself; but it is also determined by his unconscious feeling of omnipotence—the mere wish to have a difficulty disappear should be enough to dispel it.

Behind the fear of changing are qualms about changing for the worse—that is, losing one's idealized image, turning into the rejected self, becoming like everybody else, or being left by analysis an empty shell; terror of the unknown, of having to relinquish safety devices and satisfactions hitherto gained, particularly those of chasing after phantoms that promise solution; and finally a fear of being unable to change—a fear that will be better understood when we come to discuss the neurotic's hopelessness.

All these fears spring from unresolved conflicts. But because we must expose ourselves to them if we want eventually to find integration, they also stand as a hindrance to our facing ourselves. They are the purgatory, as it were, through which we must wander before we can attain salvation.

CHAPTER TEN

Impoverishment of Personality

To CONSIDER the consequences of unresolved conflicts is to enter a seemingly limitless territory and one that has been little explored. We could, perhaps, approach it by embarking on a discussion of certain symptomatic disorders like depression, alcoholism, epilepsy, or schizophrenia, hoping thereby to gain a better understanding of particular disturbances. I prefer, however, to examine it from a more general vantage point and to pose the question: What do unresolved conflicts do to our energies, our integrity, and our happiness? I adopt this approach because it is my conviction that we cannot grasp the significance of any symptomatic disorder without an understanding of its fundamental human basis. The tendency in modern psychiatry to reach for a handy theoretical formulation to account for existing syndromes is not unnatural in view of the need of the clinician whose job it is to deal with them. But to do so is as little feasible, let alone scientific, as for a construction engineer to build the top floors of a building before laying the foundation.

Some of the elements that enter into our question have already been mentioned and need only be elaborated here. Others are implicit in our previous discussions; still others will have to be added. Our aim is to leave the reader not with some vague notion that un-

resolved conflicts are injurious but to convey a fairly
clear and comprehensive picture of the havoc they inflict on the personality.

Living with unresolved conflicts involves primarily a
devastating *waste of human energies,* occasioned not
only by the conflicts themselves but by all the devious
attempts to remove them. When a person is basically
divided he can never put his energies wholeheartedly
into anything but wants always to pursue two or more
incompatible goals. This means that he will either scat-
ter his energies or actively frustrate his efforts. The
former is true of persons whose idealized image, like
Peer Gynt's, lures them into believing that they can
excel in everything. A woman, in this case, wants to be
an ideal mother, a perfect cook and hostess, dress well,
play a prominent social and political role, be a devoted
wife, have affairs outside marriage and do productive
work of her own to boot. Needless to say, this cannot be
done; she will be bound to fail in all these pursuits,
and her energies—no matter how potentially gifted she
is—will be wasted.

Of more general relevance is the frustration of a
single pursuit where incompatible motivations block
each other. A man may want to be a good friend but
be so domineering and demanding that his potentialities in this direction are never realized. Another wants
his children to get on in the world, but his drive for
personal power and his insistent rightness interfere.
Someone wants to write a book but gets a splitting
headache or is seized with a deadly fatigue whenever
he cannot immediately formulate what he wants to say.
In this instance it is again the idealized image that is

responsible: since he is the mastermind, why shouldn't brilliant thoughts flow from his pen like rabbits from a magician's hat? And when they do not, he bursts with rage at himself. Someone else may have an idea of real value that he wants to present at a meeting. But he wishes not only to express it in a way that will be impressive and put others in the shade; he also wants to be liked and to avoid antagonizing, and at the same time anticipates ridicule because of the externalization of his self-contempt. The result is that he cannot think at all and the pertinent thought he might have produced never reaches fruition. Still another could be a good organizer but by reason of his sadistic trends antagonizes everyone around him. It is hardly necessary to give further examples because all of us can find plenty of them if we look at ourselves and those about us.

There is an apparent exception to this lack of clear direction. Sometimes neurotic persons show a curious single-mindedness of purpose: men may sacrifice everything including their own dignity to their ambition; women may want nothing of life but love; parents may devote their entire interest to their children. Such persons give the impression of wholeheartedness. But, as we have shown, they are actually pursuing a mirage which appears to offer a solution of their conflicts. The apparent wholeheartedness is one of desperation rather than of integration.

It is not the conflicting needs and impulses alone that consume and dissipate energies. Other factors in the protective structure have the same effect. There is the eclipse of whole areas of the personality due to the suppression of parts of the basic conflict. The parts eclipsed are still sufficiently active to interfere, but they cannot be put to constructive use. The process thus constitutes a loss of energy that might otherwise be used for self-assertion, for co-operation, or for establishing good human relationships. There is, to mention only one other factor, the alienation from self that robs a person of his motor force. He can still be a good worker, he may even be able to make a considerable effort when put under external pressure, but he collapses when left to his own resources. This does not only mean that he cannot do anything constructive or enjoyable with his free time; it means nothing less than that all his creative forces may go to waste.

For the most part, a variety of factors combine to create large areas of diffuse inhibition. In order to understand and eventually remove a single inhibition, we usually have to come back to it again and again, tackling it from all the angles we have discussed.

Waste or misdirection of energy can stem from three major disturbances, all symptomatic of unresolved conflicts. One of these is a general *indecisiveness*. It may be prevalent in everything, from trifles to matters of greatest personal importance. There may be an endless wavering whether to eat this dish or that, whether to buy this or that suitcase, whether to go to the movies or listen to the radio. It may be impossible to decide on a career or on any step within a career; to decide between two women; to decide whether or not to get a divorce; whether to die or to live. A decision that must be made and that would be irrevocable is a real ordeal and may leave a person panic-stricken and exhausted.

Though their indecisiveness may be marked, people are often unaware of it because they unconsciously exert every effort to avoid decision. They procrastinate; they just "don't get around to" doing things; they allow themselves to be swayed by chance or else leave the decision to someone else. They may also becloud issues to a degree that leaves no basis upon which to make a decision. The aimlessness that follows from all this is likewise not usually apparent to the person himself. The many unconscious devices employed to cover up pervasive indecision account for the comparative rarity with which analysts hear complaints about what is actually a common disorder.

Another typical manifestation of divided energies is a general *ineffectualness*. I do not have in mind here an inaptitude in a particular field, which might be due to lack of training or interest in the subject. Nor is it a question of untapped energies such as William James describes in a most interesting paper [1] pointing to the fact that a reservoir of energy becomes available when one does not succumb to the first signs of fatigue, or under pressure of external circumstances. Ineffectualness in this context is that which results from a person's incapacity to exert his best efforts by reason of his inner crosscurrents. It is as if he were driving a car with the brakes on; inevitably the car is slowed down. Sometimes this is literally applicable. Everything a person attempts may be done much more slowly than either his abilities or the inherent difficulty of the task would warrant. Not that he makes insufficient effort; on the

---

[1] William James, *Memories and Studies*, Longmans, Green, 1934.

contrary, he must put an inordinate amount of effort into anything he does. It may take him hours, for instance, to write a simple report or master a simple mechanical device. What exactly impedes him of course varies. He may unconsciously rebel against what he feels as coercion; he may be driven to perfect every minute detail; he may be furious at himself—as in an example above—for not acquitting himself superbly at the first attempt. The ineffectualness does not only manifest itself in slowness; it may also appear in awkwardness or forgetfulness. A maid or a housewife will not do her work well if she secretly feels it unfair that, gifted as she is, she should be doing menial work. And her ineffectualness will usually not be confined to this particular activity but will pervade all her endeavors. From the subjective standpoint this means working under strain, with the inevitable consequence of becoming easily exhausted and needing much sleep. Any kind of work under these conditions is bound to take more out of a person, just as a car will suffer if it is driven with locked brakes.

The inner strain—and the ineffectualness as well—is present not only in work but also to a very marked degree in dealing with people. If someone wants to be friendly but at the same time resents the idea because he feels it to be ingratiating, he will be stilted; if he wants to ask for something but also feels he should command it, he will be ungracious; if he wants to assert himself but also to comply, he will be hesitant; if he wants to make contact with people but anticipates rejection, he will be shy; if he wants to have sexual relations but also wants to frustrate the partner, he will be frigid—and so on. The more pervasive the countercurrents, the greater the strain of living.

Some persons are aware of such inner strain; more often they become aware of it only if under special conditions it is increased; sometimes it strikes them only by contrast with the few occasions when they can relax, feel at ease, and be spontaneous. For the resulting fatigue they usually hold other factors responsible—a weak constitution, an overdose of work, a lack of sleep. Any of these, it is true, may play a role, but a much less significant one than is ordinarily believed.

A third symptomatic disturbance relevant here is a general *inertia*. Patients suffering from it sometimes accuse themselves of being lazy, but actually they cannot be lazy and enjoy it. They may have a conscious aversion to effort of any kind, and may rationalize it by saying that it is quite enough if they have the ideas and that it is up to others to carry out the "details"— that is, do the work. The aversion to effort may also appear as a fear that effort would be injurious to them. This fear is understandable in view of the fact that they know they tire easily; and it may be enhanced by the advice of physicians who take the exhaustion at its face value.

Neurotic inertia is a paralysis of initiative and action. Generally speaking, it is the result of a strong alienation from self and a lack of goal-direction. Long experience of strained and unsatisfactory effort leaves the neurotic with a fairly pervasive listlessness—although periods of hectic activity sometimes intervene. Of the single contributing factors the most influential are the idealized image and sadistic trends. The very fact of having to make a consistent effort may be felt by the neurotic as humiliating evidence that he is *not* his idealized image, while the prospect of doing something that might be only mediocre is so deterring that he prefers not to do it at all but perform magnificently in fantasy. The gnawing self-contempt that invariably follows from the image robs him of the assurance that he can do anything worth while, thereby burying as in quicksand all incentive and joy in activity. Sadistic trends, particularly in their repressed form (inverted sadism), make a person lean over backward from anything resembling aggression, with the result that a more or less complete psychic paralysis may ensue. General inertia is of particular significance since it covers not only action but feelings as well. The amount of energy that is wasted in consequence of unresolved neurotic conflicts is unfathomably great. Since neuroses are ultimately a product of the particular civilization, such a thwarting of human gifts and qualities stands as a serious indictment of the culture in question.

Living with unresolved conflicts entails not only a diffusion of energies but also a split in matters of a moral nature—that is, in moral principles and all the feelings, attitudes, and behavior that bear upon one's relations with others and affect one's own development. And as in the case of energies division leads to waste, so in moral questions it leads to a loss of moral wholeheartedness, or in other words to an impairment of moral integrity. Such impairment is brought about by the contradictory positions assumed as well as by the attempts to conceal their contradictory nature.

Incompatible sets of moral values appear in the basic conflict. Despite all attempts to harmonize them, all of them keep operating. This means, however, that none is or can be taken seriously. The idealized image, for all that it includes elements of true ideals, is essentially a counterfeit, and as difficult for the person himself or for the untrained observer to distinguish from the real thing as a counterfeit bank note from a valid one. The neurotic, as we have seen, may believe—in good faith—that he follows ideals, may castigate himself for every apparent lapse, thus giving an impression of overconscientiousness in pursuit of his standards; or he may intoxicate himself with thinking and talking about values and ideals. My assertion that he nevertheless does not take his ideals seriously means that *they do not have obligating power for his life*. He applies them when it is easy or useful for him to do so, while at other times he conveniently blots them out. We have seen instances of this in our discussion of blind spots and compartmentalizing—instances that would be inconceivable in the case of persons who took their ideals seriously. Nor if the ideals were genuine could they be thrown overboard as easily as they are—for instance in a person who, again in good faith, claims ardent devotion to a cause, but when exposed to temptation turns traitor.

In general, the characteristics of an impairment of moral integrity are a decrease in sincerity and an increase in egocentricity. It is interesting to note in this connection that in Zen Buddhist writings sincerity is equated with wholeheartedness, pointing to the very conclusion we reach on the basis of clinical observation

—namely, that nobody divided within himself can be wholly sincere.

MONK: I understand that when a lion seizes upon his opponent, whether it is a hare or an elephant, he makes an exhaustive use of his power; pray tell me what is this power?

MASTER: The spirit of sincerity (literally, the power of not-deceiving).

Sincerity, that is, not-deceiving, means "putting forth one's whole being," technically known as "the whole being in action" . . . in which nothing is kept in reserve, nothing is expressed under disguise, nothing goes to waste. When a person lives like this, he is said to be a golden-haired lion; he is the symbol of virility, sincerity, wholeheartedness; he is divinely human.[2]

Egocentricity is a moral problem in so far as it entails making others subservient to one's own needs. Instead of their being regarded and treated as human beings in their own right they come to be merely means to an end. They have to be appeased or liked for the sake of allaying one's own anxiety; they have to be impressed for the sake of lifting one's own self-respect; they have to be blamed because one cannot assume responsibility for oneself; they have to be defeated because of one's own need to triumph, and so on.

The particular ways in which these impairments manifest themselves vary with the individual. Most of them have already been dealt with in some other con-

[2] D. T. Suzuki, *Zen Buddhism and Its Influence on Japanese Culture*, The Eastern Buddhist Society (Kyoto), 1938.

nection and need only be reviewed here in a more systematic fashion. I shall not attempt to be exhaustive. That would be difficult, if for no other reason than that we have not yet discussed sadistic trends and must postpone doing so because they are to be regarded as an end stage of neurotic development. Starting with the most obvious, whatever course a neurosis takes, *unconscious pretenses* are always a factor. Outstanding are the following:

The pretense of love. The variety of feelings and strivings that can be covered by the term love or that are subjectively felt as such is astonishing. It may cover parasitic expectations on the part of a person who feels too weak or too empty to live his own life.[3] In a more aggressive form it may cover a desire to exploit the partner, to gain through him success, prestige, and power. It may express a need to conquer someone and to triumph over him, or to merge with a partner and live through him, perhaps in a sadistic way. It may mean a need to be admired, and so secure affirmation for one's idealized image. For the very reason that love in our civilization is so rarely a genuine affection, maltreatment and betrayal abound. We are left with the impression, then, that love turns into contempt, hate, or indifference. But love does not swing around so easily. The fact is that the feelings and strivings prompting pseudo love eventually come to the surface. Needless to say, this pretense operates in the parent-child relation and in friendship as well as in sexual relationships.

The pretense of goodness, unselfishness, sympathy,

[3] *Cf.* Karen Horney, *Self-Analysis, op. cit.,* Chapter 8, Morbid Dependency.

and the like is akin to the pretense of love. It is characteristic of the compliant type and is reinforced by a
particular kind of idealized image as well as by the
need to blot out all aggressive impulses.

The pretense of interest and knowledge is most conspicuous in those who are alienated from their emotions
and believe that life can be mastered by intellect alone.
They have to pretend that they know everything and
are interested in everything. But it appears also in a
more insidious way in persons who seem to be devoted
to a particular calling, and without being aware of it
use this interest as a steppingstone to success, power, or
material advantage.

The pretense of honesty and fairness is most frequently found in the aggressive type, especially when
he has marked sadistic trends. He sees through the pretenses of love and goodness in others and believes that
because he does not subscribe to the common hypocrisies of feigning generosity, patriotism, piety, or
whatever, he is particularly honest. Actually he has his
own hypocrisies of a different order. His lack of current
prejudices may be a blind and negativistic protest
against any traditional values. His ability to say no may
be not strength but a wish to frustrate others. His frank-
ness may be a wish to deride and humiliate. A desire
to exploit may be behind the legitimate self-interest to
which he confesses.

The pretense of suffering must be discussed in greater
detail because of the confused views that circulate
around it. Analysts who adhere strictly to Freud's theories share with the layman the belief that the neurotic
wants to feel abused, wants to worry, has a need for

punishment. The data supporting the concept that the neurotic wants to suffer are well known. But the term *wants* actually covers a variety of intellectual sins. The authors who propound the theory fail to appreciate that the neurotic suffers much more than he knows and that he usually becomes aware of his suffering only when he begins to recover. What is even more relevant, they do not seem to understand that suffering from unresolved conflicts is inevitable and entirely independent of one's personal wishes. If a neurotic lets himself go to pieces, he certainly does not bring such harm on himself because he wants it but because inner necessities compel him to do so. If he is self-effacing and offers the other cheek, he—at least unconsciously—hates doing so and despises himself for it; but he is in such terror of his own aggressiveness that he must go to the opposite extreme and let himself be abused in some way or other.

Another characteristic that has contributed to the notion of a propensity for suffering is the tendency to exaggerate or dramatize any affliction. It is true that suffering may be felt and displayed for ulterior motives. It may be a plea for attention or forgiveness; it may be unconsciously used for purposes of exploitation; it may be an expression of repressed vindictiveness and be employed then as a means to exort sanctions. But in view of the inner constellation, these are the only ways open to the neurotic to achieve certain ends. It is true also that he often lays his suffering to false causes and so gives the impression of wallowing in suffering for no good reason. Thus he may be disconsolate and attribute it to his being "guilty," while in reality he suffers from not being his idealized image. Or he may feel lost when separated from a loved one, and though he attributes his feeling to his deep love, in reality—being torn within himself—he cannot bear living alone. Finally, he may falsify his affects and believe that he suffers when actually he is filled with rage. A woman, for instance, may think she is suffering when her lover has not written at the appointed time, but is really angered because she wants things to happen exactly as she expects them or because she feels humiliated at any seeming lack of attention. Suffering, in this case, is unconsciously preferred to recognizing the rage and the neurotic drives responsible for it, and is emphasized because it serves to cover up the duplicity involved in the whole relationship. In none of these instances, however, can it be inferred that the neurotic wants to suffer. What is expressed is an unconscious pretense of suffering.

A further specific impairment is the development of *unconscious arrogance*. Again I mean this in the sense of arrogating to oneself qualities one does not have or that one has in a lesser degree than is assumed, and of unconsciously claiming the right on this ground to be demanding and derogatory toward others. All neurotic arrogance is unconscious in that the person is unaware of any false claims. The distinction here is not between conscious and unconscious arrogance but between one that is conspicuous and one that is hidden behind overmodesty and apologetic behavior. The difference lies in the measure of available aggression rather than in the measure of existing arrogance. In the one instance a person openly demands special prerogatives; in the other he is hurt if they are not spontaneously given to him. What is lacking in either case is what might be called realistic humility, that is, a recognition—not only in words but with emotional sincerity—of the limitations and imperfections of human beings in general and of one's own in particular. In my experience every patient is averse to thinking or hearing of any limitation that might apply to him. This is especially true of the patient with hidden arrogance. He would rather scold himself mercilessly for having overlooked something than admit, with St. Paul, that "our knowledge is piecemeal." He would rather recriminate himself for having been careless or lazy than admit that nobody can be equally productive at all times. The surest indication of hidden arrogance is the apparent contradiction between self-recrimination, with its apologetic attitude, and the inner irritation at any criticism or neglect from outside. It often requires close observation to discover these hurt feelings because the overmodest type is likely to repress them. But actually he may be just as demanding as the openly arrogant person. His criticism of others, too, is no less scathing, though what appears on the surface may be only a self-effacing admiration. Secretly, however, he expects the same perfection of others as of himself, which means that he lacks a true respect for the particular individuality of others.

Another moral problem is the *inability to take a definite stand* and the *undependability* that goes with it. The neurotic rarely takes a stand in accordance with the objective merits of a person, idea, or cause but rather on the basis of his own emotional needs. Since these, however, are contradictory, one position can easily be exchanged for another. Hence many neurotics are readily swayed—unconsciously bribed, as it were—by the lure of greater affection, greater prestige, recognition, power, or "freedom." This applies to all their personal relationships, whether individual or as part of a group. They often cannot commit themselves to a feeling or opinion about another person. Some unsubstantiated gossip may alter their opinion. Some disappointment or slight, or what is felt as such, may be reason enough to drop a "very good friend." Some difficulty encountered may turn their enthusiasm into listlessness. They may change their religious, political, or scientific views because of some personal attachment or resentment. They may take a stand in a private conversation but give way under the slightest pressure by some authority or group —often without knowing why they changed their opinion or even that they have done so at all.

A neurotic may unconsciously avoid obvious wavering by not making up his mind in the first place, by "sitting on the fence," leaving every alternative open. He may rationalize such an attitude by pointing to the actual intricacies of the situation, or he may be determined by a compulsive "fairness." Unquestionably a genuine striving to be fair is valuable. It is true also that a conscientious wish to be fair makes it harder to take a definite stand in many situations. But fairness can be a compulsory part of the idealized image, and its function then is to make taking a stand unnecessary, while at the same time allowing the person to feel "anointed" for being above prejudiced struggle. In this case there is a tendency to be indiscriminate in believing that two viewpoints are really not so contradictory, or that in a dispute between two persons there is right on both sides. It is a pseudo objectivity which prevents a person from recognizing the essential issues in any matter.

On this score there are great differences among various types of neuroses. The greatest integrity is to be found in those truly detached persons who have kept out of the whirlpool of neurotic competition and neurotic attachments and are not easily bribed by either "love" or ambition. Also, their onlooker attitude toward life often permits them a considerable objectivity in their judgment. But not every detached person can take a stand. He may be so averse to disputing or to committing himself that even in his own mind he takes no clear position, but either muddles issues or at best registers the good and the bad, the valid and the invalid, without arriving at any conviction of his own.

The aggressive type, on the other hand, seems to contradict my assertion that as a rule the neurotic has difficulty in taking a stand. Especially if he is inclined to rigid rightness he seems to have an unusual capacity for definite opinions, for defending them and sticking to them. But the impression is deceptive. When this type is definite it is too often because he is opinionated rather than because he has genuine convictions. Since they serve as well to choke all doubts in himself, his opinions will often have a dogmatic or even fanatic character. Moreover, he can be bribed by prospects of power or success. His dependability is restricted to the limits set by his drive for domination and recognition.

The neurotic's attitude toward *responsibility* can be confusing. This is due in part to the fact that the word

itself has a variety of implications. It may refer to con-
scientiousness in fulfilling duties or obligations.
Whether the neurotic is responsible in this sense depends on his particular character structure; it is not a
thing that all neuroses have in common. Responsibility
for others may mean feeling responsible for one's own
actions in so far as they affect someone else; but it may
also be a euphemism for dominating others. Holding
oneself responsible when it implies taking blame may
be merely an expression of rage at not being one's idealized image and in this sense have nothing to do with
responsibility.

If we ourselves are clear as to exactly what is meant
by taking responsibility for oneself, we will understand
that it is hard, if not impossible, for any neurotic to
assume it. It means in the first place to acknowledge
in a matter-of-fact way—to oneself and others—that such-
and-such were one's intentions, one's words or one's
actions, and to be willing to take the consequences. This
would be the opposite of lying or of putting the blame
on others. To take responsibility for himself in this
sense would be hard for the neurotic because as a rule
he does not know what he is doing or why he is doing
it and has a keen subjective interest in not knowing.
That is why he often tries to wriggle out by denying,
forgetting, belittling, inadvertently supplying other
motivations, feeling misunderstood, or getting confused.
And since he tends to exclude or absolve himself, he
readily assumes that his wife, his business partner, his
analyst are responsible for any difficulty that arises. Another factor that frequently contributes to his inability
to take the consequences of his actions or even to see

them is a hidden feeling of omnipotence, on the basis of which he expects to do whatever he pleases and get away with it. To recognize the inescapable consequences would shatter this feeling. A final factor that is relevant here looks at first glance like an intellectual incapacity to think in terms of cause and effect. The neurotic commonly gives the impression of being inherently able to think only in terms of fault and punishment. Almost every patient feels that the analyst is blaming him, whereas actually the analyst is only confronting him with his difficulties and their consequences. Outside the analytical situation he may feel like a culprit always under suspicion and attack and therefore constantly on the defensive. In reality this is an externalization of intrapsychic processes. As we have seen, the source from which these suspicions and attacks stem is his own idealized image. It is this inner process of fault finding and defense, plus its externalization, that makes it almost impossible for him to conceive of a cause-and-effect relation where he himself is concerned. But where difficulties of his own are not involved he can be just as matter-of-fact as anyone else. If the streets get wet because it is raining he does not ask whose fault it is but accepts the causal connection.

When we speak of assuming responsibility for the self we mean, in addition, the capacity to stand up for what we believe is right and a willingness to take the consequences if our action or decision should prove to be wrong. This, too, is difficult when a person is divided by conflicts. For which of the conflicting trends within himself should he or could he stand up? None of them represents what he really wants or believes in. He really could stand up only for his idealized image. This, how-ever, does not permit of the possibility of being wrong. Hence if his decision or action leads to trouble, he must falsify matters and ascribe the adverse conse-quences to someone else.

A comparatively simple example will illustrate this problem. A man at the head of an organization craves unlimited power and prestige. Nothing may be done or decided without him; he cannot bring himself to dele-gate functions to others who by virtue of their particular training might be better equipped to handle certain affairs. There is, in his own mind, nothing he does not know best. Besides, he does not want anyone else to feel or to become important. His expectations of himself would be impossible to measure up to if only because of limitations of time and energy. But this particular man wants not only to dominate; he is also compliant and needs to be superhumanly good. As a result of his unresolved conflicts he has all the earmarks we have described—inertia and need for sleep, indecision and procrastination, and hence cannot organize his time. And since he feels the keeping of appointments as in-tolerable coercion, he secretly enjoys making people wait. In addition, he does many unimportant things merely because they flatter his vanity. Finally, his urge to be a devoted family man consumes much of his time and thought. Naturally, then, things do not function very well in the organization; but seeing no flaw in himself, he puts the blame on others or on untoward circumstances.

Again let us ask, for which part of his personality could he take responsibility? For his tendency to domi-

nate, or for his tendency to comply, appease, and
ingratiate himself? To begin with, he is unaware of
either. But even if he were aware of them he could not
uphold one and discard the other, because both are
compulsory. Furthermore, his idealized image does not
allow him to see anything in himself but ideal virtues
and unlimited capacities. Hence he cannot take responsibility for the consequences that inevitably follow from
the operation of his conflicts. To do so would bring into
clear relief all that he is so anxious to conceal from
himself.

Generally speaking, the neurotic is especially averse
—unconsciously—to assuming responsibility for the consequences of his actions. He shuts his eyes to even the
very obvious ones. Unable to do away with his conflicts,
he insists—again unconsciously—that he, all powerful
as he is, should be able to cope with them. Consequences, he believes, may catch up with others, but for
him they do not exist. He must therefore keep on dodg-
ing any recognition of the laws of cause and effect. If
he would only open his mind to them they could teach
him a powerful lesson. They demonstrate in a fool-
proof way that his system of living does not work, that
for all his unconscious cunning and trickery he cannot
budge the laws that operate in our psychic life with the
same inexorability as in the physical sphere.[4]

As a matter of fact, the whole subject of responsibility
has little appeal for him. He sees—or dimly senses—only

[4] *Cf.* Lin Yutang, *Between Tears and Laughter, op. cit.* In the
chapter on "Karma," the author expresses his astonishment at
the lack of understanding of these psychic laws in Western civilization.

its negative aspects. What he does not see, and learns to appreciate only gradually, is that by turning his back on it he defeats his ardent strivings for independence. He hopes to attain independence by defiantly excluding all commitments, whereas in reality the assuming of responsibility for oneself and to oneself is an indispensable condition of real inner freedom.

In order not to recognize that his problems and his suffering stem from his inner difficulties, the neurotic resorts to any of three devices—and often to all of them. Externalization may be applied to the hilt at this point, in which case everything from food, climate, or constitution to parents, wife, or fate is blamed for the particular calamity. Or he may take the attitude that since nothing is his fault it is unfair that any misfortune should befall him. It is unfair that he should fall ill, get old, or die, that he should be unhappily married, have a problem child, or that his work remain unrecognized. This kind of thinking, which may be conscious or unconscious, is doubly wrong, for it eliminates not only his own share in his difficulties but also all the factors independent of himself that have a bearing on his life. Nevertheless, it has a logic of its own. It is the typical thinking of an isolated being who is centered exclusively upon himself and whose egocentricity makes it impossible for him to see himself as only a small link in a greater chain. He simply takes it for granted that he should derive all the good of living at a particular time in a particular social system, but resents being linked with others for good or ill. Therefore he cannot see why he should suffer from anything in which he has not been personally implicated.

The third device is connected with his refusal to recognize cause-and-effect relationships. Consequences appear in his mind as isolated occurrences, unrelated to himself or his difficulties. A depression or a phobia, for instance, may seem to descend upon him from the blue. This, of course, might be due to psychological ignorance or lack of observation. But in analysis we can see that the patient offers a most tenacious resistance to taking cognizance of any impalpable connections. He may remain incredulous or forget them; or he may feel that the analyst, instead of speedily removing the troublesome disturbances—which was what he came for—puts the "blame" on him and cleverly saves his own face. Thus a patient may have become familiar with factors relevant to his inertia but close his mind to the obvious fact that his inertia slows up not only his analysis but everything else he does. Or another may have become aware of his aggressive-derogatory behavior toward people but cannot understand why he often has quarrels and is disliked. That these difficulties exist within him is one thing, but his actual day-to-day problems are something else again. This separation of his inner troubles from their effect on his life is one of the mainsprings of the whole tendency to compartmentalize.

Resistance toward recognizing the consequences of neurotic attitudes and drives is for the most part deeply concealed and may be easily overlooked by the analyst for the very reason that to him the connection is so obvious. This is unfortunate, because unless the patient is made aware that he blinds himself to consequences and the reasons for which he does so, he cannot possibly realize to what an extent he interferes with his own life. Awareness of consequences is the most powerful curative factor in analysis in that it impresses on the patient's mind that only by changing certain things within himself can he ever attain freedom.

If, then, the neurotic cannot be held accountable for his pretenses, his arrogance, his egocentricity, his shirking of responsibility, can we speak in terms of morals at all? The argument will be raised that, as physicians, we need only be concerned with the patient's illness and cure, and that his morals are not our province. It will be pointed out that one of Freud's great merits was to have overthrown the "moralistic" attitude I seem to advocate!

Such arguments are deemed scientific; but are they tenable? Can we really exclude in matters of human behavior judgments as to right and wrong? If analysts decide what needs analytical examination and what does not, do they not really proceed on the basis of the very judgments they consciously reject? There is a danger, however, in such implicit judgments: they are likely to be made on either too subjective or too traditional a ground. Thus an analyst may feel that a man's philandering need not be analyzed, while a woman's deserves scrutiny. Or if he believes in an unbridled living out of sexual drives, he may decide that faithfulness, whether in a man or a woman, needs analysis. Actually, judgments should be made on the basis of the particular patient's neurosis. The question to be decided is whether an attitude the patient has assumed has consequences injurious to his development and to his relations with people. If it has, it is wrong and needs to be tackled. The reasons for the analyst's conclusions should be explicitly stated to the patient in order to enable him to make up his own mind in the matter. And finally, do not the above arguments contain the same fallacy as exists in the patient's thinking—namely, that morals are only a question of judgment and not primarily one of fact coupled with consequences? Let us take neurotic arrogance as an example. It exists as a fact no matter whether the patient is responsible for it or not. The analyst believes that arrogance is a problem for the patient to recognize and eventually to overcome. Does he assume this critical attitude because he has learned in Sunday school that arrogance is sinful and humility a virtue? Or is his judgment determined by the fact that arrogance is unrealistic and has adverse consequences, the burden of which is inevitably the patient's—again regardless of his responsibility. The consequences, though, in the case of arrogance bar the patient from knowing himself, and so thwart his development. Also, the arrogant patient is apt to be unfair to others, and this again has its repercussions—not merely in subjecting him to occasional clashes with others but in alienating him from people generally. This, however, only drives him deeper into his neurosis. Because the patient's morals in part result from his neurosis and in part contribute to its maintenance, the analyst has no choice but to be interested in them.

CHAPTER ELEVEN

Hopelessness

DESPITE his conflicts a neurotic can be contented at times, can enjoy things to which he feels himself attuned. But his happiness is dependent upon too many conditions for it to be of frequent occurrence. He will not take pleasure in anything unless, for instance, he is alone—or unless he shares it with someone else; unless he is the dominating factor in the situation—or unless he is approved of on all sides. His chances are further narrowed by the fact that the conditions for happiness are so often contradictory. He may be glad to have another person take the lead but he may at the same time resent it. A woman may enjoy her husband's success but she may also envy him for it. She may enjoy giving a party but have to have everything so perfect that she is exhausted before it begins. And when the neurotic does find temporary happiness, it is all too easily disturbed by his manifold vulnerabilities and fears.

Moreover, mishaps of the sort that occur in every life assume undue proportions in his mind. Any minor failure may plunge him into a depression because it proves his general unworthiness—even when it is due to factors beyond his control. Any harmless critical remark may set him worrying or brooding, and so on. As a result he is ordinarily more unhappy and discontented than the circumstances warrant.

This situation, bad enough as it stands, is aggravated by a further consideration. Human beings can apparently endure an amazing amount of misery as long as there is hope; but neurotic entanglements invariably generate a measure of hopelessness, and the more severe the entanglements the greater the hopelessness. It may be deeply buried: superficially the neurotic may be preoccupied with imagining or planning conditions that would make things better. If only he were married, had a larger apartment, a different foreman, a different wife; if only she were a man, a little older or younger, a little taller or not so tall—then everything would be all right. And sometimes the elimination of certain disquieting factors really does prove helpful. More often, however, such hopes merely externalize inner difficulties and are doomed to disappointment. The neurotic expects a world of good from external changes, but inevitably carries himself and his neurosis into each new situation.

Hope that rests on externals is naturally more preva-lent among the young; that is one of the reasons why an analysis of a very young person is less simple than one might expect. As people grow older and one hope after another fades, they are more willing to take a good look at *themselves* as a possible source of distress.

Even when a general feeling of hopelessness is unconscious, its existence and its strength can be inferred from sundry indications. There may be episodes in the life history that show the person's reaction to disappointments to have been of an intensity and duration wholly disproportionate to the provocation. Thus one may encounter a complete hopelessness resulting apparently from unrequited love in adolescence. from betrayal by a friend, unjust dismissal from a job, failure in examinations. Naturally one would first try to fathom whatever special reasons there might be for so profound a reaction. But over and above any special reasons, it will usually be found that the unfortunate experience drains a much deeper well of hopelessness. Similarly, a preoccupation with death or the ready emergence of suicidal thoughts—with or without affect—point to a pervasive hopelessness, even though the person presents a façade of optimism. A general flippancy, a refusal to take anything seriously—whether in the analytical situation or outside it—is another indication, as is easy discouragement in the face of difficulty. Much of what Freud has defined as negative therapeutic reaction belongs here. A new insight which, though it may be painful, offers a way out may only provoke discouragement and an unwillingness to go through the hardship of again working through a new problem. Sometimes this looks as though the patient did not trust himself to overcome the particular difficulty; but in reality it expresses his lack of hope of ever being able to gain by it. Under these conditions it is only logical for him to complain that the particular insight hurts or frightens him and to resent being upset by the analyst. A preoccupation with foreseeing or foretelling the future is also a sign of hopelessness. Although on the surface this looks like an anxiety about life in general, about being caught unawares, about making mistakes, it will be observed that in such cases the outlook is invariably tinged with pessimism. Like Cassandra, many neurotics foresee largely evil, rarely good. This focusing on the dark side of life rather than on the bright should make one sus-

pect a deep personal hopelessness, no matter how in-
telligently it is rationalized. Finally, there is the chronic
depressed condition, which can be so hidden and insidious that it does not strike one as depression. Persons
so afflicted may function fairly well. They can be pleas-
ant and have a good time, but it may take them hours
to rouse themselves in the morning, to come to life, as
it were, to put up with life again. Life is so permanent
a burden that they hardly feel it as such and do not
complain about it. But their spirits are permanently at
a low ebb.

While the sources of hopelessness are always unconscious, the feeling itself can be fairly conscious. A person may have a pervasive sense of doom. Or he may
take a resigned attitude toward life in general, expecting nothing good, feeling simply that life must be en-
dured. Or he may express it in philosophical terms, saying in effect that life is essentially tragic and only fools
deceive themselves about man's unalterable fate.

Already in the preliminary interview one may get
an impression of the patient's hopelessness. He will be
unwilling to make the smallest sacrifice, to undergo
even a minor inconvenience, to take the slightest risk.
He may give the appearance then of being too self-
indulgent. But the fact is that he sees no compelling
reason to make sacrifices when he expects to gain nothing from them. Similar attitudes can be seen outside
analysis. People remain in thoroughly unsatisfactory
situations which with a bit of effort and initiative could
be bettered. But a person may be so completely paralyzed by his hopelessness that moderate difficulties
seem to him insurmountable obstacles.

Sometimes a chance remark will bring this condition to the surface. A patient may respond to the analyst's simply saying that a certain problem is not yet solved and requires more work with the question: "You don't think it is hopeless?" And when he becomes aware of his despair he usually cannot account for it. He will be likely to ascribe it to various external factors, ranging from his job or his marriage to the political situation. But it is not due to any concrete or temporary circumstance. He feels hopeless about ever making anything of his life, ever being happy or free. He feels forever excluded from all that could make his life meaningful.

Perhaps Søren Kierkegaard has given the most profound answer. In *The Sickness unto Death* [1] he says that all despair is fundamentally a despair of being ourselves. Philosophers of all times have stressed the pivotal significance of being ourselves and the despair attendant on feeling barred from its approximation. It is the central theme of Zen Buddhist writings. Among modern authors I quote only John Macmurray: [2] "What other significance can our existence have than to be ourselves fully and completely?"

Hopelessness is an ultimate product of unresolved conflicts, with its deepest root in the despair of ever being wholehearted and undivided. A mounting scale of neurotic difficulties leads to this condition. Basic is the sense of being caught in conflicts like a bird in a net, with no apparent possibility of ever extricating

[1] Søren Kierkegaard, *op. cit.*
[2] John Macmurray, *Reason and Emotion,* Appleton-Century, 1938.

oneself. On top of this come all the attempts at solution which not only fail but increasingly alienate the person from himself. Repetitive experience serves to intensify the hopelessness—talents that never lead to achievement, whether because again and again energies are scattered in too many directions or because the difficulties arising in any creative process are enough to deter the person from further pursuit. This may apply as well to love affairs, marriages, friendships, which are shipwrecked one after another. Such repeated failures are as disheartening as is the experience of laboratory rats when, conditioned to jump into a certain opening for food, they jump again and again only to find it barred.

There is, furthermore, the factually hopeless enterprise of trying to measure up to the idealized image. It is hard to say whether this may not be the most potent of the factors producing hopelessness. There is no question, however, that in analysis hopelessness comes into full relief when the patient becomes aware that he is far from being the uniquely perfect person he sees in his imagination. He feels hopeless at such a time not only because he despairs of ever attaining those fantastic heights but even more because he responds to this realization with profound self-contempt, detrimental to the expectation of ever attaining anything, whether in love or in work.

Final among the contributing factors are all the processes that cause a person's center of gravity to shift from within himself and that make him cease to be the active propellant in his life. The outcome of it all is that he loses faith in himself and in his development as a human being; he tends to give up—an attitude which, although it may pass unnoticed, is in its consequences grave enough to be called a psychic death. As Kierkegaard [3] says: "But despite the fact [of his despair] . . . he may nevertheless . . . be perfectly well able to live on, to be a man, as it seems, to occupy himself with temporal things, get married, beget children, win honor and esteem—and perhaps no one notices that in a deeper sense he lacks a self. About such a thing as that not much fuss is made in the world; for a self is a thing the world is least apt to inquire about, and the thing of all things the most dangerous for a man to let people notice that he has it. The greatest danger, that of losing one's own self, may pass off as quietly as if it were nothing; every other loss, that of an arm, a leg, five dollars, a wife, etc., is sure to be noticed."

From my experience in supervisory work I know that the problem of hopelessness is often not clearly envisaged by the analyst and hence not properly dealt with. Some of my colleagues have been so overwhelmed by the patient's hopelessness—which they recognized but did not see as a problem—that they became hopeless themselves. This attitude is of course fatal to an analysis, for no matter how good the technique or how brave the effort, the patient senses that the analyst has really given him up. The same holds true outside the analytical situation. Nobody can be a constructively helpful friend or mate who does not believe in the possibility of the companion's fulfilling his own potentialities.

Sometimes colleagues have made the opposite mistake of not taking the patient's hopelessness seriously enough.

[3] Søren Kierkegaard, *op. cit.*

They felt the patient needed encouragement and gave it—which is commendable, but quite insufficient. When this happens, the patient, even if he appreciates the analyst's good intentions, is quite justified in being annoyed with him, since deep down he knows that his hopelessness is not just a mood that can be dissipated by well-meant encouragement.

In order to take the bull by the horns and tackle the problem directly, it is necessary first to recognize from indirect indications like the ones cited above that the patient feels hopeless and the extent to which he feels so. Then it must be understood that his hopelessness is fully warranted by his entanglements. The analyst must realize and explicitly convey to the patient that his situation is hopeless only so long as the status quo persists and is regarded as unchangeable. In simplified form, the whole problem is illustrated by a scene from Chekhov's *Cherry Orchard*. The family, faced with bankruptcy, are in despair at the thought of leaving their estate with its beloved cherry orchard. A man of affairs offers the sound suggestion that they build small houses for rent on a part of the estate. With their hidebound views, they cannot countenance such a project, and since there is no other solution they remain without hope. They ask helplessly, as if they had not heard the suggestion, whether nobody can advise or help them. If their mentor were a good analyst he would say: "Of course the situation is difficult. But what makes it hopeless is your own attitude toward it. If you would consider changing your claims on life there would be no need to feel hopeless."

The belief that the patient can really change, which

means essentially that he can really resolve his conflicts, is the factor that determines whether or not the therapist dare to tackle the problem and whether he can do it with a reasonable chance of success. It is here that my differences with Freud come into clear relief. Freud's psychology and the philosophy underlying it are essentially pessimistic. This is patent in his outlook on the future of mankind [4] as well as in his attitude toward therapy.[5] And on the basis of his theoretical premises, he cannot be anything but pessimistic. Man is driven by instincts which at best are only to be modified by "sublimation." His instinctual drives for satisfaction are inevitably frustrated by society. His "ego" is helplessly tossed about between instinctual drives and the "superego," which itself can only be modified. The superego is primarily forbidding and destructive. True ideals do not exist. The wish for personal fulfillment is "narcissistic." Man is by nature destructive and a "death instinct" compels him either to destroy others or to suffer. All these theories leave little room for a positive attitude toward change and limit the value of the potentially splendid therapy Freud originated. In contrast, I believe that compulsive trends in neuroses are not instinctual but spring from disturbed human relationships; that they can be changed when these improve and that conflicts of such origin can really be resolved. This does not mean that therapy based on the principles

[4] Sigmund Freud, "Civilization and its Discontents," *International Psychoanalytical Library*, Vol. XVII, Leonard and Virginia Woolf, 1930.
[5] Sigmund Freud, "Analysis Terminable and Interminable," *International Journal of Psychoanalysis*, 1937.

I advocate has no limitations. Much work remains to be done before we can clearly determine these limitations. But it does mean that we have well-founded reasons for believing in the possibility of radical change.

Why, then, is it so important to recognize and tackle a patient's hopelessness? In the first place, this approach is of value in dealing with special problems like depressions and suicidal tendencies. We can, it is true, lift an individual depression by merely uncovering the particular conflicts in which the person is caught at the time, without touching upon his general hopelessness. But if we want to prevent recurring depressions it has to be tackled because it is the deeper source from which the depressions emanate. Nor can insidious chronic depression be coped with unless one goes to this original source.

The same holds true for suicidal conditions. We know that such factors as acute despair, defiance, and vindictiveness lead to suicidal impulses; but it is often too late to prevent suicide after the impulse has become manifest. By paying minute attention to the less dramatic signs of hopelessness and by taking up the problem with the patient at the proper time, it is probable that many suicides could be averted.

Of more general significance is the fact that the patient's hopelessness constitutes a hindrance to the cure of any severe neurosis. Freud was inclined to call everything that hampered a patient's progress *resistance*. But we could hardly regard hopelessness in this light. In analysis we have to deal with a counterplay of retarding and forward-moving forces, with resistance and incentive. Resistance is a collective term for all the forces within the patient that operate to maintain the status quo. His incentive, on the other hand, is produced by the constructive energy that urges him on toward inner freedom. This is the motive power with which we work and without which we could do nothing. It is the force that helps the patient overcome resistance. It makes his associations productive, thereby giving the analyst a chance for better understanding. It gives him the inner strength to endure the inevitable pain of maturing. It makes him willing to take the risk of abandoning attitudes that have given him a feeling of safety and to make the leap into the unknown of new attitudes to-ward himself and others. The analyst cannot drag the patient through this process; the patient himself must want to go. It is this invaluable force that is paralyzed by a condition of hopelessness. And in failing to recognize and tackle it the analyst deprives himself of his best ally in the battle against the patient's neurosis.

The patient's hopelessness is not a problem that can be solved by any single interpretation. There is already a substantial gain if, instead of being engulfed by a feeling of doom that he regards as unalterable, the patient begins to recognize it as a problem that may eventually be solved. This step liberates him sufficiently to go ahead. There will, of course, be ups and downs. He may feel optimistic, even overoptimistic, if he acquires some helpful insight, only to succumb to his hopelessness again as soon as he approaches a more upsetting one. Each time the matter must be tackled anew. But the hold it has on the patient will relax as he realizes that he can really change. His incentive will grow accordingly. It may be limited, at the beginning of the analysis, to a mere wish to get rid of his most disturbing symptoms. But it gains strength as the patient becomes increasingly aware of his shackles, and as he gets a taste of how it feels to be free.

CHAPTER TWELVE

Sadistic Trends

PERSONS in the grip of neurotic hopelessness manage to "carry on" in one way or another. If their capacity to be creative has not been too greatly damaged by their neurosis they may be able fairly consciously to resign themselves to the state of their personal lives and concentrate on a field in which they can be productive. They may submerge themselves in a social or religious movement or in the work of an organization. Their work may be useful; the fact that they lack zest can be outweighed by their having no personal ax to grind.

Others, in adapting themselves to their particular frame of life, may cease to question it but yet not attach much meaning to it, trying merely to fulfill their obligations. John Marquand depicts this kind of life in *So Little Time*. It is, I believe, the state that Erich Fromm [1] describes as a "defect" condition, in contrast to neurosis. I interpret it, however, as the outcome of neurotic processes.

They may, on the other hand, give up all serious or promising pursuits and turn to the periphery of life, trying to snatch from it some bit of enjoyment, finding their interest in a hobby or in incidental pleasures like good eating, convivial drinking, minor sexual affairs.

[1] Erich Fromm, "Individual and Social Origins of Neurosis," *American Sociological Review*, Vol. IX, No. 4, 1944.

Or they may drift and deteriorate, let themselves go to pieces. Unable to do any consistent work, they take to drink, gambling, whoring. The kind of alcoholism described by Charles Jackson in *The Lost Week-End* would represent an end stage of such a condition. In this connection it might be interesting to examine whether an unconscious determination to go to pieces may not supply a powerful psychic contribution to such chronic diseases as tuberculosis and cancer.

Finally, persons without hope may turn destructive, but at the same time make an attempt at restitution by living vicariously. This, in my opinion, is the meaning of sadistic trends.

Because Freud regarded sadistic trends as instinctual, psychoanalytical interest has been largely focused on the so-called sadistic perversions. Sadistic patterns in everyday relationships, though not ignored, have not been strictly defined. Any kind of assertive or aggressive behavior is conceived of as a modification or sublimation of instinctual sadistic trends. Freud, for instance, regarded a striving for power as such a sublimation. It is true that a striving for power can be sadistic; but in a person who sees life as a battle of all against all, it can merely represent a struggle for survival. Actually, it need not be neurotic at all. The result of this lack of discrimination is that we have neither a comprehensive picture of the forms sadistic attitudes may take nor any criteria as to precisely what is sadistic. It is left pretty much to individual intuition to determine what may rightly be called sadism and what may not—a situation hardly conducive to sound observation.

The mere act of hurting others is in itself no indication of a sadistic tendency. A man may be engaged in a struggle of a personal or general nature in the course of which he has to hurt not only his adversaries but his associates as well. Hostility toward others may also be merely reactive. A person can feel hurt or frightened and want to hit back with a force that, while disproportionate to the objective provocation, is subjectively quite in keeping with it. It is easy, however, to deceive oneself on this score: all too often a justifiable reaction is claimed when actually a sadistic tendency was in operation. But the difficulty in distinguishing one from the other does not mean that reactive hostility is nonexistent. Finally, there are all those offensive tactics of the aggressive type who feels he is fighting for survival. I should not call any of these aggressions sadistic; others may get hurt in the process, but the hurting or damaging is an inevitable by-product rather than a prime intention. To put it simply, we could say that although the kinds of action we refer to here are aggressive or even hostile, they are not perpetrated in a mean spirit. There is no conscious or unconscious satisfaction derived from the very fact of hurting.

In contrast, let us consider some typical sadistic attitudes. We can best observe these in persons who are fairly uninhibited in expressing their sadistic tendencies toward others, whether they themselves are conscious of having such tendencies or not. When, in the following, I speak of a sadistic person, I mean a person whose attitudes toward others are predominantly sadistic.

Such a person may want to *enslave* others or to enslave the partner in particular. His "victim" must be a superman's slave, a creature not only without wishes, feelings, or initiative of his own but without any claims whatever upon the master. This tendency may take the form of molding or educating the victim, as Professor Higgins in *Pygmalion* molds Eliza. At best it can have some constructive aspects, as in the case of parents with children or teachers with pupils. Occasionally this aspect obtains in sexual relations, particularly if the sadistic partner is the more mature. It is sometimes conspicuous in homosexual relations between an older and a younger man. But even there the devil's horns will show themselves if the slave gives any indication of meaning to go his own way, of having friends or interests of his own. Frequently, though not invariably, the master is haunted by a possessive jealousy and uses it as a means of torture. It is peculiar to sadistic relationships of this kind that keeping a hold over the victim is *of more absorbing interest than the person's own life.* He will neglect his career, forego the pleasures or advantages of meeting other persons rather than grant the partner any independence.

The ways in which the partner is kept enslaved are characteristic. They vary only within a comparatively limited range and depend on the personality structure of both members. The sadistic person will give the partner just enough to make the relationship appear worth his while. He will fulfill certain of the partner's needs —though rarely more than will keep him at a minimum subsistence level, psychically speaking. And he will impress upon him the unique quality of what he gives. Nobody else, he will point out, could give him such understanding, such support, so much sexual satisfaction or so many interests; nobody else, indeed, would

ever put up with him. Again, he may hold him with the
lure of better times—implicitly or explicitly, he will
promise love or marriage or a better financial status or
better treatment. Sometimes he will stress his own need
of the partner and appeal to him on that ground. All
these tactics are the more effective in that by being so
possessive and so disparaging he isolates the partner
from others. If the latter is made sufficiently dependent
he may finally threaten to leave him. Still further means
of intimidation may be employed, but these have so
much a life of their own that they will be discussed
separately, in another context. Naturally, we cannot
understand what goes on in such a relationship without
taking into account the characteristics of the partner.
Often he is of the compliant type and hence in dread
of desertion; or he may be a person who has profoundly
repressed his own sadistic drives and is helpless on that
account—as will be shown later.

The mutual dependence that accrues from such a situation arouses resentment not only in the enslaved but
in the enslaver as well. If the latter's need for detachment is pronounced, he is especially resentful of the
partner's absorbing so much of his thought and energy.
Not realizing that he himself has created these cramping
ties, he may reproach the partner for being grasping
or clinging. His wanting to break away on such occasions is as much an expression of fear and resentment as
a means of intimidation.

Not all sadistic craving aims at enslavement. Another
sort finds its satisfaction in *playing on the emotions*
of another person as on an instrument. In his novel,
Diary of the Seducer, Søren Kirkegaard shows how a

man *who expects nothing of his own life* can be entirely
absorbed by the game itself. He knows when to show
interest and when to be indifferent. He is hypersensitive in anticipating and observing the girl's reactions
to him. He knows what will arouse and what will check
her erotic desires. But his sensitivity is limited to the
requirements of the sadistic play: he is totally uncon-
cerned with what this experience might mean to the
girl's life. What in Kirkegaard's novel is conscious
shrewd calculation, more often goes on unconsciously.
But it is the same game of attracting and rejecting,
charming and disappointing, elevating and degrading,
bringing joy and bringing grief.

A third characteristic is to *exploit* the partner. Exploitation is not necessarily a sadistic enterprise; it may
be employed merely for the sake of gain. In sadistic
exploitation, too, gain may be a consideration, but it is
often illusory and wholly out of proportion to the affect
put into its pursuit. For the sadist, exploitation becomes
a kind of passion in its own right. What matters is to
experience the triumph of getting the better of others.
Its specifically sadistic coloring appears in the means
used for exploitation. The partner is subjected, directly
and indirectly, to ever mounting demands, and is made
to feel guilty or humiliated if he does not fulfill them.
The sadistic person can always find a justification for
feeling discontented or unfairly treated, and for demanding still more on that account. Ibsen's *Hedda
Gabler* illustrates how the fulfilling of such demands
never evokes gratitude, and how the demands themselves are often prompted by the desire to hurt the other
person and put him in his place. They may have to do

with material things or sexual needs or aid in establishing a career; they may be demands for special consideration, exclusive devotion, boundless tolerance. There is nothing specifically sadistic in their content: what does point to sadism is the expectation that the partner should, by whatever means are available, fill out a life that is emotionally empty. This, too, is well illustrated by Hedda Gabler in her constant complaints of feeling bored and wanting stimulation and excitement. The need to feed, vampirelike, on the emotional vitality of another person is as a rule completely unconscious. But it is probable that it is at the bottom of the craving to exploit and that it is the soil from which the expressed demands draw their sustenance.

The nature of the exploitation becomes still clearer when we realize that there is simultaneously a tendency to *frustrate* others. It would be a mistake to say that the sadistic person never wants to give anything. Under certain conditions he may even be generous. What is typical of sadism is not a niggardliness in the sense of withholding but a much more active, though unconscious, impulse to thwart others—to kill their joy and to disappoint their expectations. Any satisfaction or buoyancy of the partner's almost irresistibly provokes the sadistic person to spoil it in some way. If the partner looks forward to seeing him, he tends to be sullen. If the partner wants sexual intercourse, he will be frigid or impotent. He may not even have to do, or fail to do, anything positive. By simply radiating gloom he acts as a depressant. To quote Aldous Huxley: [2] "He did

[2] Aldous Huxley, *Time Must Have a Stop*, Harper and Brothers, 1944.

not have to do anything: it was enough for him just to *be*. They shriveled and turned black by mere infection." And a little later: "What an exquisite refinement of the will to power, what an elegant cruelty! And what an amazing gift for that contagious gloom which damps even the highest spirits and stifles the very possibility of joy."

As significant as any of these is the sadistic person's tendency to *disparage* and *humiliate* others. He is remarkably keen at seeing shortcomings, at discovering the weak spots in others and pointing them out. He knows intuitively where others are sensitive and can be hurt. And he tends to use his intuition mercilessly for derogatory criticism. This may be rationalized as honesty or as a wish to be helpful; he may believe himself to be sincerely troubled by doubts in regard to the other person's competence or integrity—but he will become panicky if the sincerity of his doubts is questioned. It may also appear as mere suspiciousness. The patient may say: "If only I could trust that person!" But after having translated him in his dreams into everything loathsome from a cockroach to a rat, how could he expect to trust him! In other words, suspiciousness can be merely a consequence of disparaging another person in one's own mind. And if the sadistic person is unaware of his disparaging attitude he may be conscious only of the resulting suspiciousness. Again it would seem more appropriate to speak of a passion for fault-finding than of simply a tendency. He not only turns his searchlight on actual flaws but is extremely adept at externalizing his own faults and so building up a case against the other fellow. If, for instance, he has upset someone by his own behavior, he will immediately show concern or even contempt for that person's emotional instability. If the partner, being intimidated, is not entirely frank with him, he will reproach him for his secrecy or for lying. He will reproach him for being dependent on him when he himself has done all he could to make him so. Such undermining is not just a matter of words but is accompanied by all sorts of scornful behavior. Humiliating and degrading sexual practices can be one of its expressions.

When any of these drives is frustrated, or when the tables are turned and the sadistic person feels himself dominated, exploited, or scorned, he may have spells of an almost insane rage. In his imagination, then, no torture is great enough to inflict upon the offender: he may kick him, beat him, slice him to pieces. These spells of sadistic rage can in turn be repressed, and give rise to a state of acute panic or some functional somatic disturbance pointing to an increase of inner tension.

What, then, is the meaning of these trends? What are the inner necessities that compel a person to behave with such cruelty? The assumption that sadistic trends are the expression of a perverted sexual drive has no basis in fact. It is true that they can be expressed in sexual behavior. In this they are no exception to the general rule that all our character attitudes are bound to manifest themselves in the sexual sphere—as they do in our way of working, in our gait, in our handwriting. It is also true that many sadistic pursuits are carried on with a certain excitement or, as I have said repeatedly, with an absorbing passion. The conclusion, however, that these affects of thrill or excitement are sexual in nature, even when they are not felt as such, merely rests on the premise that every excitement is in itself sexual. But there is no evidence to substantiate such a premise. Phenomenologically the two sensations of sadistic thrill and sexual abandon are entirely different in nature.

The assertion that sadistic impulses are a persisting infantile trend has a certain appeal in that young children are often cruel to animals or younger children, and apparently get a thrill out of it. In view of this superficial similarity one might say that the elementary cruelty of the child has merely been refined. But actually it is not only refined: the cruelty of the adult sadist is different in kind. As we have seen, it has distinct characteristics which are lacking in the child's outright cruelty. The child's cruelty seems to be a comparatively simple response to feeling oppressed or humiliated. He asserts himself by exercising his vengeance on weaker folk. Specifically sadistic trends are more complicated and grow from more complicated roots. Besides, like every attempt to account for later peculiarities by relating them directly to early experiences, this one, too, leaves an all-important question unanswered: What are the factors that account for the persistence and elaboration of the cruelty?

Each of the above hypotheses fastens upon only a single aspect of sadism—sexuality in the one case, cruelty in the other—and fails to account even for these characteristics. The same can be said of an explanation offered by Erich Fromm,[3] though it comes closer to the

[3] Erich Fromm, *Escape from Freedom,* Farrar and Rinehart, 1941.

essentials than do the others. Fromm points out that the sadistic person does not want to destroy the one to whom he attaches himself, but because he cannot live his own life must use the partner for a symbiotic existence. This is definitely true, but it still does not sufficiently explain why a person is compulsively driven to tamper with the lives of others, or why the tampering takes the particular forms that it does.

If we regard sadism as a neurotic symptom, we must start, as always, not by trying to explain the symptom but by seeking to understand the structure of the personality that develops it. When we approach the problem from this angle we recognize that nobody develops pronounced sadistic trends who has not a profound feeling of futility as regards his own life. Poets intuitively sensed this underlying condition long before we were able to dig it out with our prodding clinical scrutiny. In the case of both Hedda Gabler and the Seducer, the possibility of ever making something of themselves or their lives was a more or less closed issue. If under these circumstances a person cannot find his way to resignation, he of necessity becomes utterly resentful. He feels forever excluded, forever defeated.

Hence he starts to hate life and all that is positive in it. But he hates it with the burning envy of one who is withheld from something he ardently desires. It is the bitter, begrudging envy of a person who feels that life is passing him by. "Lebensneid," Nietzsche called it. He does not feel that others have their sorrows, too: "they" sit at the table while he goes hungry; "they" love, create, enjoy, feel healthy and at ease, belong somewhere. The happiness of others and their "naïve" expectations of pleasure and joy irritate him. If he cannot be happy and free, why should they be so? In the words of Dostoevski's Idiot, he cannot forgive them their happiness. He must trample on the joy of others. His attitude is illustrated by the story of the teacher doomed by tuberculosis who spits on his pupil's sandwiches and is elated at his power to crush them. That was a conscious act of vindictive envy. In the sadist the tendency to frustrate and to crush the spirit of others is as a rule deeply unconscious. But the purpose is the same sinister one as that of the teacher: to impart his suffering to others; if others are as defeated and degraded as he, his own misery is tempered in that he no longer feels himself the only one afflicted.

Another way he alleviates his gnawing envy is by a "sour grapes" tactic, mastered to such perfection that even the trained observer is easily deceived by it. As a matter of fact, his envy is so deeply buried that he himself would deride any suggestion of its existence. His focusing upon the painful, burdensome, or ugly side of life is thus not only an expression of his bitterness but even more of his interest in proving to himself that he is not missing anything. His constant faultfinding and devaluating stem in part from this source. He will take note, for instance, of the one part of a beautiful woman's body that is not perfect. Coming into a room, his eyes will be arrested by the one color or piece of furniture that does not match the rest. He will pick out the one flaw in an otherwise good speech. Similarly, whatever is wrong in other persons' lives or in their characters or in their possible motivations will loom large in his mind. If he is sophisticated he will ascribe this attitude to his being sensitive to imperfections. But the fact is that he turns his searchlight on these alone, leaving everything else in the dark.

Although he succeeds in assuaging his envy and discharging his resentment, his devaluating attitude in turn gives rise to a permanent feeling of disappointment and discontent. If he has children, for instance, he thinks primarily of the burdens and obligations that go with them; if he has no children he feels that this most important human experience has been denied him. If he has no sexual relations he feels deprived and is concerned about the dangers of continence; if he has sexual relations he feels humiliated by them and ashamed of them. If he has an opportunity to make a trip, he chafes under the inconveniences; if he cannot travel he deems it a disgrace to have to stay at home. Since it does not occur to him that the sources of his chronic discontent could lie within himself, he feels entitled to impress upon others how they fail him and to make ever greater demands whose fulfillment can never satisfy him.

The bitter envy, the tendency to devaluate and the resulting discontent account to some extent for certain of the sadistic trends. We understand why the sadist is driven to frustrate others, to inflict suffering, to find fault, to make insatiable demands. But we can appreciate neither the extent of his destructiveness nor his arrogant self-righteousness until we consider what his hopelessness does to his relation to himself.

While he violates the most elementary requirements of human decency, he at the same time harbors within

himself an idealized image of particularly high and
rigid moral standards. He is one of those (we have
spoken of them before) who, despairing of ever being
able to measure up to such standards, have consciously
or unconsciously resolved to be as "bad" as possible. He
may succeed in being "bad" and wallow in it with a
kind of desperate delight. But by doing so the chasm
between the idealized image and the actual self becomes
unbridgeable. He feels beyond repair and beyond forgiveness. His hopelessness becomes deeper and he develops the recklessness of a person who has nothing to
lose. As long as this condition persists it is factually impossible for him to assume a constructive attitude toward himself. Any direct attempt to make him constructive is doomed to futility and betrays ignorance of
his condition.

His self-loathing reaches such dimensions that he
cannot take a look at himself. He must fortify himself
against it by reinforcing an already existing armor of
righteousness. The slightest criticism, neglect, or absence of special recognition can mobilize his self-
contempt and so must be rejected as unfair. He is
compelled, therefore, to externalize his self-contempt, to
blame, berate, humiliate others. This, however, throws
him into the toils of a vicious circle. The more he despises others the less is he aware of his self-contempt—
and the self-contempt grows more violent and merciless the more hopeless he becomes. To strike out against
others is then a matter of self-preservation. The process
is illustrated by the example cited previously of the patient who accused her husband of indecision and

wanted to tear herself to pieces when she realized that
she was really furious at her own indecision.

In this light we begin to appreciate why it is imperative for the sadistic person to disparage others. And
we can see now, too, the inner logic of his compulsive
and often fanatical drive to reform others, or at least to
reform the partner. Since he himself cannot measure
up to his idealized image, the partner must do so; and
the merciless rage he feels toward himself is vented on
the partner for any failure in this direction. He may
ask himself sometimes: "Why don't I leave him alone?"
But it is apparent that such rational considerations are
of no avail as long as the inner battle persists and is externalized. He usually rationalizes the pressure he exerts
on the partner as "love" or interest in the partner's
"development." Needless to say, it is not love. But
neither is it an interest in the partner's development
along his own lines, in accordance with his own inner
laws. In reality he tries to enforce upon the partner
the impossible task of realizing his—the sadist's—idealized image. The righteousness which he had to develop
as a shield against self-contempt permits him to do so
with smug assurance.

An understanding of this inner struggle provides us
also with a better insight into another more general factor inherent in sadistic symptoms: the vindictiveness
that often seeps through every cell of the sadist's personality like a poison. He is and must be vindictive because he turns his violent contempt for himself outward. Since his righteousness prevents him from seeing
his share in any difficulty that arises he must feel that
he is the one who is abused and victimized; since he

cannot see that the source of all his despair lies within himself he must hold others responsible for it. They have ruined his life, they have to make up for it—they have to take what's coming to them. It is this vindictiveness, more than any other factor, that kills within him all feelings of sympathy and mercy. Why should he have sympathy for those who have spoiled his life—and in addition are better off than he? In individual instances the desire for revenge may be conscious; he may be aware of it, for example, in reference to his parents. He is not aware, however, that it is a pervasive character trend.

The sadistic person, as we have seen him thus far, is one who because he feels excluded and doomed runs amok, venting his rage at others in blind vindictiveness. And we understand, now, that by making others miserable he seeks to alleviate his own misery. But this can hardly be the whole explanation. The destructive aspects alone do not explain the absorbing passion characteristic of so many sadistic pursuits. There must be some more positive gains, gains that for the sadistic person are of vital importance. This statement might seem to contradict the assumption that sadism is an outgrowth of hopelessness. How can a hopeless person hope for something and go after it, what is more, with such consuming energy? The fact is, however, that from a subjective standpoint there is considerable to be gained. In degrading others he not only allays his intolerable self-contempt but at the same time gives himself a feeling of superiority. When he molds the lives of others he not only gains a stimulating feeling of power over them but also finds a substitute meaning for his life. When he exploits others emotionally he provides a vicarious emotional life for himself that lessens his own sense of barrenness. When he defeats others he wins a triumphant elation which obscures his own hopeless defeat. This craving for vindictive triumph is probably his most intense motivating force.

All his pursuits serve as well to gratify his hunger for thrills and excitement. A healthy, well-balanced person does not need such thrills. The more mature he is the less does he care for them. But the emotional life of the sadistic person is empty. Almost all feelings except those of anger and triumph have been choked off. He is so dead that he needs these sharp stimuli to feel alive.

Last but not least, his sadistic dealings with others provide him with a feeling of strength and pride which reinforce his unconscious feeling of omnipotence. During analysis a patient's attitude toward his sadistic trends undergoes profound changes. When he first becomes aware of them, he is likely to assume a critical attitude toward them. But his implied rejection is not wholehearted; it is rather a matter of giving lip service to current standards. Intermittently he may have spells of self-loathing. At a later period, however, when he is on the verge of relinquishing his sadistic way of living, he may suddenly feel that he is about to lose something precious. He may then for the first time consciously experience elation at being able to do with others as he pleases. He may express concern lest analysis turn him into a contemptible weakling. And again, as so often in analysis, the patient's concern is subjectively warranted: bereft of his power to make others serve his

emotional needs he sees himself as a wretched and helpless creature. In time he will realize that the feeling of
strength and pride he derived from being sadistic is a
poor substitute. It was precious to him only because
real strength and real pride were unattainable.

When we are aware of the nature of these gains we
see that there is no contradiction in the statement that
a hopeless person may be frantically searching for something. But it is not greater freedom or greater self-
fulfillment that he expects to find: all that goes to make
up his hopelessness remains unchanged, and he does
not count on changing it. What he pursues are substitutes.

The emotional gains are achieved by living vicariously. *To be sadistic means to live aggressively and for
the most part destructively, through other persons.* But
this is the only way a person so utterly defeated can live.
The recklessness with which he pursues his goals is the
recklessness born of despair. Having nothing to lose, he
can only gain. In this sense sadistic strivings have a
positive goal and must be regarded as an *attempt at
restitution.* The reason why the goal is so passionately
pursued is that in triumphing over others the sadistic
person is able to remove his own abject sense of defeat.

The destructive elements inherent in these strivings
cannot, however, remain without repercussions on the
individual himself. We have already pointed to the
heightening of self-contempt. An equally significant re-
percussion is the generation of anxiety. This is in part
a fear of retaliation: he fears that others will treat him
as he treats them—or wants to treat them. Consciously,

it appears not so much as a fear as in simply taking it for granted that they would "give him a raw deal" if they could—that is, if he does not prevent it by being constantly on the offensive. He must be so alert in foreseeing and forestalling any possible attack that for all practical purposes he will be inviolable. The unconscious conviction of his own inviolability often plays a considerable role. It gives him a lordly feeling of security: *he* could never be hurt, he could never be exposed, he could never have an accident or contract a disease; he could not, indeed, ever die. If nonetheless he does get hurt, by persons or circumstances, his pseudo security is shattered and he is likely to be seized by acute panic.

In part, his anxiety is a fear of the explosive, destructive elements within himself He feels like a person who carries a highly charged bomb around with him. Excessive self-control and continuous vigilance are needed to keep these dangerous elements in check. They may come to the surface when he drinks, if he is not too frightened to loosen up under the influence of liquor. He may then become violently destructive. The impulses may also come closer to awareness under special conditions that for him represent temptation. Thus the sadist in Zola's *Bête Humaine* becomes panicky when attracted by a girl because this arouses an impulse to murder her. Witnessing an accident or any act of cruelty may bring on a seizure of fear because these awaken his own impulse to destroy.

These two factors—self-contempt and anxiety—are largely responsible for the repression of sadistic impulses. The thoroughness and depth of repression vary.

en the destructive impulses are merely kept from
reness. By and large it is astonishing how much
sadistic behavior can be lived out without the individual's knowing it. He is conscious only of occasional desires to mistreat a weaker person, of being excited when
he reads about sadistic acts, or of having some obviously
sadistic fantasies. But these sporadic glimpses remain
isolated. The bulk of what he does to others in his daily
behavior is for the most part unconscious. His numbness of feeling for himself and others is one factor that
blurs the issue; until this is dispelled he cannot emotionally experience what he does. Besides, the justifica-
tions brought to bear to conceal the sadistic trends are
often clever enough to deceive not only the sadistic person himself but even those affected by them. We must
not forget that sadism is an end stage of a severe neurosis. Hence the kind of justification employed will
depend upon the structure of the particular neurosis
from which the sadistic trends stem. The compliant
type, for instance, will enslave the partner under the
unconscious pretense of love. His demands will be attributed to his needs. Because he is so helpless or so
apprehensive or so ill, the partner should do things for
him. Because he cannot be alone, the partner should
always be with him. His reproaches will be expressed
indirectly by his demonstrating, unconsciously, how
much others make him suffer.

The aggressive type expresses sadistic trends quite
undisguisedly—which, however, does not mean that he
is any more aware of them. He has no hesitation in
showing his discontent, his scorn, and his demands but
feels that, besides being entirely justified, he is simply

being frank. He will also externalize his lack of regard for others and the fact that he exploits them, and will intimidate them by telling them in no uncertain terms how much they abuse him.

The detached person is singularly unobtrusive in expressing sadistic trends. He will frustrate others in a quiet way, making them feel insecure by his readiness to withdraw, conveying the impression that they are cramping or disturbing him, and taking secret delight in letting them make fools of themselves.

But sadistic impulses can be much more deeply repressed, and then give rise to what might be called an inverted sadism. What happens here is that the person so greatly fears his impulses that he leans over backward to keep them from being revealed to himself or others. He will shun everything that resembles assertion, aggression, or hostility and as a result will be profoundly and diffusely inhibited.

A brief outline will give an idea of what this process entails. To lean over backward from enslaving others is to be incapable of giving any order, much less of assuming a position of responsibility or leadership. It makes for overcaution in exerting influence or giving advice. It involves the repression of even the most legitimate jealousy. A good observer will merely notice that the person gets a headache, a stomach ailment, or some other symptom when things do not go his way.

Leaning over backward from exploiting others brings self-effacing tendencies to the fore. It shows in not daring to express any wish—not daring even to have a wish; in not daring to rebel against abuse or even to feel abused; in tending to regard the expectations or demands of others as better justified or more important than one's own; in preferring to be exploited rather than assert one's own interest. Such a person is between the devil and the deep blue sea. He is frightened of his impulses to exploit but despises himself for his unassertiveness, which he registers as cowardice. And when he is exploited—as will naturally happen—he is caught in an unsolvable dilemma and may react with a depression or some functional symptom.

Similarly, instead of frustrating others he will be overanxious not to disappoint them, to be considerate and generous. He will go to great lengths to avoid anything that could conceivably hurt their feelings or in any way humiliate them. He will intuitively find something "nice" to say—an appreciative remark, for instance, that will heighten their self-confidence. He tends automatically to take blame on himself and will be profuse in his apologies. If he must make a criticism he will make it in the mildest possible form. Even when others grossly abuse him he will show nothing but "understanding." But at the same time he is hypersensitive to humiliation and suffers excruciatingly under it.

The sadistic play on emotions, when deeply repressed, may give place to a feeling that one is powerless to attract anyone. Thus a person may honestly believe—often in spite of good evidence to the contrary—that he is unattractive to the opposite sex, that he has to content himself with the crumbs. To speak in this case of a feeling of inferiority is merely to use another word for what the person is conscious of anyhow, and what may simply be an expression of his self-contempt.

But of relevance here is the fact that the notion of un-
attractiveness may be an unconscious recoil from the
temptation of playing the exciting game of conquering
and rejecting. During analysis it may gradually become
clear that the patient has unconsciously falsified the
whole picture of his love relations. And a curious
change will take place: the "ugly duckling" becomes
aware of his desire and capacity to attract people, but
turns against them with indignation and contempt as
soon as they take his advances seriously.

The consequent personality picture is deceptive and
difficult to evaluate. Its similarity to the compliant type
is striking. As a matter of fact, while the overtly sadistic
person ordinarily belongs to the aggressive type, the
inverted sadist began, as a rule, by developing predominantly compliant trends. The likelihood is that he
was especially hard hit and crushed into submission in
childhood. He may have falsified his feelings, and, instead of rebelling against the oppressor, turned to loving him. As he grew older—perhaps around puberty—
the conflicts became unbearable and he took refuge in
detachment. But when confronted with failure he could
no longer stand the isolation of his ivory tower. He
then seemingly reverted to his former dependence, but
with this difference: his need for affection became so
desperate that he was willing to pay any price *not* to be
left alone. At the same time his chances of finding affection were diminished because his need for detachment—
which was still present—constantly interfered with his
desire to attach himself to someone. Worn out by this
struggle, he became hopeless and developed sadistic
tendencies. But his need for people was so insistent that

he had not only to repress his sadistic trends but to lean over backward to conceal them.

Being with others is, in this event, a strain—though he may not realize it. He tends to be stilted and shy. He must constantly play a role that is contrary to his sadistic impulses. It is only natural that he himself should think he is really fond of people; and it comes as a shock to him when in analysis he wakes up to the fact that he has very little feeling for them at all, or at least is quite uncertain what his feelings are. At this point he is inclined to take this apparent lack for an unalterable fact. But actually he is merely in process of relinquishing his pretense of positive feelings, and unconsciously prefers to feel nothing rather than face his sadistic impulses. A positive feeling for others can only begin to develop when he recognizes those impulses and starts to overcome them.

There are certain elements in the picture, however, that to the trained observer will indicate the presence of sadistic trends. To begin with, there is always some insidious way in which he can be seen to intimidate, exploit, and frustrate others. There is usually a perceptible though unconscious contempt for others, superficially attributed to their lower moral standards. In addition, there are a number of incongruities which point to sadism. The person, for instance, may sometimes put up with sadistic behavior directed at himself with apparently limitless patience but at other times show hypersensitivity to the slightest domination, exploitation, or humiliation. Finally, he gives the impression of being "masochistic"—namely, of indulging in feeling victimized. But since the term and the concept behind it are misleading, it is better to steer away from it and describe instead the elements involved. Being pervasively inhibited in asserting himself, the inverted sadist will in any case be readily abused. But, in addition, because he chafes under his own weakness, he is often actually attracted to openly sadistic persons, at once admiring and abhorring them—just as the latter, sensing in him a willing victim, are attracted to him. Thus he puts himself in the way of exploitation, frustration, and humiliation. Far from enjoying such maltreatment, however, he suffers under it. What it gives him is an opportunity to live out his own sadistic impulses through someone else, without having to face his own sadism. He can feel innocent and morally indignant—while hoping at the same time that some day he will get the better of the sadistic partner and triumph over him.

Freud observed the picture I describe but vitiated his findings with unwarranted generalizations. In fitting them into the frame of his whole philosophy, he took them as proof that no matter how good a person is on the surface, he is inherently destructive. Actually, the condition is a particular outgrowth of a particular neurosis.

We have come a long way from the point of view that regards a sadistic person as a sexual pervert or that uses elaborate terminology to say he is mean and vicious. The sexual perversions are comparatively rare. When they are present they are merely one expression of a general attitude toward others. The destructive trends are undeniable; but when we understand them we see a suffering human being behind the apparently inhuman behavior. With this we open the possibility of reaching such a human being by therapy. We find him a desperate individual who seeks restitution for a life that has defeated him.

Conclusion: Resolution of Neurotic Conflicts

THE MORE we realize what infinite harm neurotic conflicts inflict on the personality, the more stringent appears the need truly to resolve them. But since, as we now understand, this cannot be done by rational decision nor by evasion nor by the exertion of will power, how can it be done? There is only one way: the conflicts can be resolved only by changing those conditions within the personality that brought them into being.

This is a radical way, and a hard one. In view of the difficulties involved in changing anything within ourselves, it is quite understandable that we should scour the ground for short cuts. Perhaps that is why patients—and others as well—so often ask: Is it enough if one sees one's basic conflict? The answer is clearly, no.

Even when the analyst—discerning quite early in the analysis just how the patient is divided—is able to help him to recognize this split, the insight is of no immediate profit. It may bring a certain relief in that the patient begins to see a tangible reason for his troubles instead of simply being lost in a mysterious haze; but he cannot apply it to his life. A perception of how his divergent parts operate and interfere with one another makes him no less divided. He hears these facts as one hears a strange message; it seems plausible, but he cannot realize its implications for himself. He is bound to invalidate it by manifold unconscious mental reservations. Unconsciously he will insist that the analyst is exaggerating the magnitude of his conflicts; that he would be quite all right if it were not for outside circumstances; that love or success would rid him of his distress; that he can evade his conflicts by keeping away from people; that though it may be true of ordinary folk that they cannot serve two masters, he with his unlimited powers of will and intelligence could manage to do so. Or he may feel—again unconsciously—that the analyst is a charlatan or a well-meaning fool, feigning professional cheerfulness; that he ought to know the patient is ruined beyond repair—which means that the patient responds to the analyst's suggestions with his own feeling of hopelessness.

Since such mental reservations point to the fact that the patient either clings to his particular attempts at solution—these being much more real to him than the conflicts themselves—or that he fundamentally despairs of recovery, all the attempts and all their consequences must be worked through before the basic conflict can profitably be tackled.

The search for an easier road has given rise to another question, lent weight by Freud's emphasis on genesis: Is it enough to relate these conflicting drives—once they have been recognized—to their origins and early manifestations in the childhood situation? Again the answer is, no—and again, for the most part, the same reasons apply. Even the most detailed recollection of his early experiences gives the patient little beyond a more lenient, more condoning attitude toward himself. It in no way makes his present conflicts any less disrupting.

A comprehensive knowledge of early environmental

influences and the changes they effected in the child's personality, though it has little direct therapeutic value, does have a bearing on our inquiry into the conditions under which neurotic conflicts develop.[1] It was, after all, the changes in his relations with himself and others that originally brought about the conflicts. I have described this development in previous publications [2] as well as in the earlier chapters of this book. Briefly, a child may find himself in a situation that threatens his inner freedom, his spontaneity, his feeling of security, his self-confidence—in short the very core of his psychic existence. He feels isolated and helpless, and as a result his first attempts to relate himself to others are determined not by his real feelings but by strategic necessities. He cannot simply like or dislike, trust or distrust, express his wishes or protest against those of others, but has automatically to devise ways to cope with people and to manipulate them with minimum damage to himself. The fundamental characteristics that evolve in this way may be summarized as an alienation from the self and others, a feeling of helplessness, a pervasive apprehensiveness, and a hostile tension in his human relations that ranges from general wariness to definite hatred.

As long as these conditions persist, the neurotic cannot possibly dispense with any of his conflicting drives.

[1] As is generally recognized, this knowledge is also of great prophylactic value. If we know what environmental factors are helpful to a child's development and what factors retard it, a way is opened to the prevention of the rank growth of neuroses in future generations.

[2] *Cf.* Karen Horney, *New Ways in Psychoanalysis, op. cit.,* Chapter 8, and *Self-Analysis, op. cit.,* Chapter 2.

On the contrary, the inner necessities from which they stem become even more stringent in the course of the neurotic development. The fact that the pseudo solutions increase the disturbance in his relations with others and with himself means that a real solution becomes less and less attainable.

The goal of therapy, therefore, can only be to change the conditions themselves. The neurotic must be helped to retrieve himself, to become aware of his real feelings and wants, to evolve his own set of values, and to relate himself to others on the basis of his feelings and convictions. If we could achieve this by some magic, the conflicts would be dispelled without their having even to be touched upon. As there is no magic, we must know what steps have to be taken to bring about the desired change.

Since every neurosis—no matter how dramatic and seemingly impersonal the symptoms—is a character disorder, the task of therapy is to analyze the entire neurotic character structure. Hence the more clearly we can define this structure and its individual variations, the more precisely can we delineate the work to be done. If we conceive of neurosis as a protective edifice built around the basic conflict, the analytical work can roughly be divided into two parts. One part is to examine in detail all the unconscious attempts at solution that the particular patient has undertaken, together with their effect on his whole personality. This would include studying all the implications of his predominant attitude, his idealized image, his externalization, and so on, without taking into consideration their specific relationship to the underlying conflicts. It would be misleading to assume that one cannot understand and work at these factors before the conflicts have come into focus, for although they have grown out of the need to harmonize the conflicts, they have a life of their own, carrying their own weight and wielding their own power.

The other part covers the work with the conflicts themselves. This would mean not only bringing the patient to an awareness of their general outline but helping him to see how they operate in detail—that is, how his incompatible drives and the attitudes that stem from them interfere with one another in specific instances: how, for example, a need to subordinate himself, reinforced by inverted sadism, hinders him from winning a game or excelling in competitive work, while at the same time his drive to triumph over others makes victory a compelling necessity; or how asceticism, stemming from a variety of sources, interferes with a need for sympathy, affection, and self-indulgence. We would have to show him also how he shuttles between extremes: how, for instance, he alternates between being overstrict with himself and overlenient; or how his externalized demands upon himself, reinforced perhaps by sadistic drives, clash with his need to be omniscient and all-forgiving, and how in consequence he wavers between condemning and condoning everything the other fellow does; or how he veers between arrogating all rights to himself and feeling he has no rights at all.

This part of the analytical work would encompass, furthermore, the interpretation of all the impossible fusions and compromises the patient is trying to make, such as trying to combine egocentricity with generosity, conquest with affection, domination with sacrifice. It would include helping him to understand exactly how his idealized image, his externalization, and so on have served to spirit away his conflicts, to camouflage them and to mitigate their disruptive force. In sum, it entails bringing the patient to a thorough understanding of his conflicts—their general effect on his personality and their specific responsibility for his symptoms.

On the whole, the patient offers a different sort of resistance in each of these sections of analytical work. While his attempts at solution are being analyzed he is bent on defending the subjective values inherent in his attitudes and trends, and so fights any insight into their real nature. During the analysis of his conflicts he is primarily interested in proving that his conflicts are not conflicts at all, and therefore blurs and minimizes the fact that his particular drives are really incompatible.

As to the *sequence* in which subjects should be tackled, Freud's advice is and probably always will be of foremost significance. Applying to analysis principles valid in medical therapy, he stressed the importance of two considerations in any approach to the patient's problems: an interpretation should be profitable, and it should not be harmful. In other words the two questions an analyst must have in mind are: Can the patient stand a particular insight at this time? and, Is an interpretation likely to have meaning for him and to set him thinking in a constructive way? What we still lack are tangible criteria of precisely what a patient can

stand and what is conducive to stimulating constructive insight. The structural differences from one patient
to another are too great to permit of any dogmatic pre-
scriptions in regard to the timing of interpretations,
but we can take as a guide the principle that certain
problems cannot be tackled profitably and without undue risk until particular changes have taken place in
the patient's attitudes. On this basis we can point to
a few measures that are invariably applicable:

It is useless to confront a patient with any major conflict as long as he is bent on pursuing phantoms that
to him mean salvation. He must see first that these pursuits are futile and interfere with his life. In highly
condensed terms, the attempts at solution should be
analyzed prior to the conflicts. I do not mean that any
mention of conflicts should be assiduously avoided.
How cautious the approach needs to be depends on the
brittleness of the whole neurotic structure. Some patients may be thrown into a panic if their conflicts are
pointed out to them prematurely. For others it will
have no meaning, will simply slide off without making
any impression. But logically one cannot expect the
patient to have any vital interest in his conflicts as long
as he clings to his particular solutions and unconsciously counts on "getting by" with them.

Another subject to be broached gingerly is the idealized image. It would lead us too far afield to discuss
here the conditions under which certain aspects of it
can be tackled at a fairly early stage. Caution is ad-
visable, however, since the idealized image is often the
only part of the patient that is real to him. It may be,
what is more, the only element that provides him with

a kind of self-esteem and that keeps him from drowning in self-contempt. The patient must have gained a measure of realistic strength before he can tolerate any undermining of his image.

To work at sadistic trends at an early period in the analysis is sure to be unprofitable. The reason lies, in part, in the extreme contrast these trends present to the idealized image. Even at a later period awareness of them often fills the patient with terror and disgust. But there is a more precise reason for postponing this piece of analysis until the patient has become less hopeless and more resourceful: he cannot possibly be interested in overcoming his sadistic trends while he is still unconsciously convinced that vicarious living is the only thing left to him.

The same guide to the timing of interpretations can be employed when its individual application depends upon the particular character structure. For example, with a patient in whom aggressive trends predominate —one who despises feelings as a weakness and acclaims everything that gives the appearance of strength—this attitude with all its implications must be worked through first. It would be a mistake to give precedence to any aspect of his need for human intimacy, no matter how obvious this need was to the analyst. The patient would resent any move of this kind as a threat to his security. He would feel that he must be on his guard against the analyst's wish to make him a "goody-goody." Only when he is much stronger will he be able to tolerate his tendencies toward compliance and self-effacement. With this patient one would also have to steer clear for some time of the problem of hopelessness, since he would be likely to resist admitting any such feeling. Hopelessness for him would have the connotation of loathsome self-pity and mean a disgraceful confession of defeat. Conversely, if compliant trends predominate, all the factors involved in "moving toward" people must be thoroughly worked through before any dominating or vindictive tendencies can be tackled. Again, if a patient sees himself as a great genius or a great lover, it would be a complete waste of time to approach his fear of being despised and rejected, and even more futile to tackle his self-contempt.

Sometimes the scope of what can be tackled at the beginning is very limited. This is so in particular when a high degree of externalization is combined with a rigid self-idealization—a position that will countenance no flaws. If certain signs reveal this condition to the analyst, he will save much time by avoiding all interpretations that even remotely imply that the source of the patient's trouble lies within himself. However, it may be feasible at this period to touch on particular aspects of the idealized image, such as the inordinate demands the patient makes upon himself.

Familiarity with the dynamics of the neurotic character structure also helps the analyst to grasp more quickly and more concisely just what the patient wants to express by his associations and hence what ought to be dealt with at the moment. He will be able to visualize and predict from seemingly insignificant indications one whole aspect of the patient's personality, and so can direct his attention to the elements to watch for. His position would be like that of the internist who, when he learns that a patient is coughing, perspiring at night, and fatigued in the late afternoon, considers the possibility of pulmonary tuberculosis and is guided accordingly in his examination.

If, for instance, a patient is apologetic in his behavior, is ready to admire the analyst, and reveals self-effacing tendencies in his associations, the analyst will visualize all the factors involved in "moving toward" people. He will examine the possibility of this being the patient's predominant attitude; and if he finds further evidence he will try to work at this from every possible angle. Similarly, if a patient repeatedly talks of experiences in which he felt humiliated, and indicates that he looks upon the analysis in this light, the analyst will know that he has to tackle the patient's fear of humiliation. And he will select for interpretation that source of the fear which at the time is most accessible. He may be able, for example, to connect it with the patient's need for affirmation of his idealized image, provided parts of the image have already come to awareness. Again, if the patient shows inertia in the analytical situation and talks of feeling doomed, the analyst will have to tackle his hopelessness in so far as that is possible at the moment. If this should occur at the very beginning he may be able only to point out its meaning—namely, that the patient has given himself up. He will then try to convey to him that his hopelessness does not spring from a factually hopeless situation but constitutes a problem to be understood and eventually solved. If the hopelessness appears at a later period the analyst may be able to relate it more specifically to his despair of finding a way out of his conflicts or of ever measuring up to his idealized image.

The suggested measures still leave ample room for the analyst's intuition and for his sensitivity to what is going on in the patient. These remain valuable, even indispensable tools which the analyst should strive to develop to his utmost. But the fact that intuition is employed does not mean that the procedure lies merely in the realm of "art" or that it is one where the application of common sense suffices. A knowledge of the neurotic character structure makes the deductions based upon it strictly scientific and enables the analyst to conduct the analysis in an exact and responsible fashion.

Nevertheless, because of the infinite individual variations in the structure, the analyst can sometimes proceed only by trial and error. When I speak of error I do not refer to such gross mistakes as imputing motivations that are alien to the patient or a failure to grasp his essential neurotic drives. What I have in mind is the very common error of making interpretations that the patient is not yet ready to assimilate. While gross mistakes are avoidable, the error of making premature interpretations is and always will be unavoidable. We can, however, reach a more speedy recognition of such errors if we are extremely alert to the way in which a patient reacts to an interpretation and are guided accordingly. It seems to me that too much emphasis has been placed on the fact of the patient's "resistance"— on his acceptance or rejection of an interpretation—and too little on exactly what his reaction signifies. This is unfortunate, because it is the kind of reaction in all its detail that indicates what has to be worked through before the patient will be ready to handle the problem the analyst has pointed out.

The following instance may serve as an illustration.
A patient realized that in his personal relationships he
showed profound irritation in response to any claim the
partner made upon him. Even the most legitimate requests were regarded as coercion and the most merited
criticisms as insults. At the same time he felt free to
demand exclusive devotion and to express his own criticisms quite frankly. He realized, in other words, that he
accorded himself every privilege while denying the partner any. It became clear to him that this attitude was
bound to mar, if not destroy, his friendships as well as
his marriage. Up to this point he had been very active
and productive in his analytical work. But the session
after he became aware of the consequences of his attitude was pervaded by silence; the patient was mildly
depressed and anxious. The few associations that did
appear pointed to a strong tendency to withdraw, which
was in decided contrast to his eagerness in previous
hours to establish a good relationship with a woman.
The impulse to withdraw was an expression of how intolerable the prospect of mutuality was to him: he accepted the idea of equality of rights in theory, but in
practice he rejected it. While his depression was a reaction to finding himself in an unsolvable dilemma,
the tendency to withdraw meant he was groping for a
solution. When he recognized the futility of withdraw-
ing, and saw that there was no way out but to change
his attitude, he became interested in the question of
why mutuality was so unacceptable to him. The associations that appeared immediately thereafter indicated
that emotionally he saw only the alternative of having
all rights or no rights whatever. He voiced an appre-

hension that if he should concede any rights he would never be able to do what he wanted but would invariably have to comply with the wishes of others. This in turn opened up the whole field of his compliant and self-effacing trends which, although they had hitherto been touched upon, had never been seen in their full depth and significance. For a number of reasons his compliance and dependence were so great that he had had to build up the artificial defense of arrogating all rights exclusively to himself. To abandon the defense at a time when his compliance was still a stringent inner necessity would have meant to submerge himself as an individual. Before he could even consider a change in his arbitrary settlement the compliant trends had to be worked through.

It will be clear from everything that has been said throughout this book that one can never exhaust a problem through a single approach; it must be returned to again and again from various angles. This is because any single attitude springs from a variety of sources and assumes new functions in the course of the neurotic development. Thus, for instance, the attitude of placating and "putting up" with too much is originally part and parcel of the neurotic need for affection and must be tackled when that need is being dealt with. Its scrutiny must be resumed when the idealized image is in question. In that light placating will be seen as an expression of the patient's notion that he is a saint. That it also involves a need to avoid friction will be understood when his detachment is under discussion. Again, the compulsive nature of the attitude will become clearer when the patient's fear of others and his need to lean over backward from his sadistic impulses come into view. In other instances a patient's sensitivity to coercion may be seen first as a defensive attitude stemming from his detachment, then as a projection of his own craving for power, and later perhaps as an expression of externalization, inner coercion, or other trends.

Any neurotic attitude or conflict that crystallizes during analysis must be understood in its relation to the personality as a whole. This is what is called working through. It involves the following steps: bringing to the patient's awareness all the overt and hidden manifestations of the particular trend or conflict, helping him to recognize its compulsive nature, and enabling him to attain an appreciation both of its subjective value and its adverse consequences.

The patient, when he discovers a neurotic peculiarity, tends to avoid examining it by immediately raising the question: "How did it come about?" Whether or not he is aware of doing so, he hopes to solve the particular problem by turning to its historical origin. The analyst must hold him back from this escape into the past and encourage him to examine first what is involved—in other words, to become familiar with the peculiarity itself. He must get to know the specific ways in which it manifests itself, the means he uses to cover it up, and his own attitudes toward it. If, for instance, the patient's dread of being compliant has become clear, he must see the extent to which he resents, dreads, and despises in himself any form of self-effacement. He must recognize the checks he has unconsciously instituted to the end of eliminating from his life all possibilities of compliance and everything involved in compliant tendencies. He will understand, then, how attitudes apparently divergent all serve this one purpose; how he has numbed his sensitivity to others to the point of being unaware of their feelings, desires, or reactions; how this has made him highly inconsiderate; how he has choked off any feeling of fondness for others as well as any desire to be liked by them; how he disparages tender feelings and goodness in others; how he tends automatically to refuse requests; how in personal relationships he feels entitled to be moody, critical, and demanding but denies the partner any of these prerogatives. Or, if it is the patient's feeling of omnipotence that has come into focus, it is not enough that he realizes that he has this feeling. He must see how from morning till night he sets impossible tasks for himself; how, for instance, he thinks he should be able to write a brilliant paper on a complex subject at top speed; how he expects himself to be spontaneous and scintillating in spite of his exhaustion; how in analysis he expects to solve a problem the moment he catches a glimpse of it.

Next, the patient must recognize that he is driven to act in accordance with the particular trend, regardless of—and often contrary to—his own desires or best interests. He must realize that the compulsion operates indiscriminately, usually without reference to factual conditions. He must see, for example, that his faultfinding attitude is turned toward friends and enemies alike; that he upbraids the partner no matter how the latter behaves: if the partner is amiable, he suspects him of feeling guilty about something; if he asserts himself, he is domineering; if he gives in, he is a weakling; if he likes to be with him, he is too easily available; if he refuses anything, he is stingy, and so on. Or if the attitude under discussion is the patient's uncertainty of being wanted or welcome, he must realize that the attitude persists despite all evidence to the contrary. Understanding the compulsive nature of a trend also involves recognizing reactions to its frustration. If, for instance, the trend that has emerged concerns the patient's need for affection, he would have to see that he feels lost and frightened at any sign of rejection or diminished friendliness, no matter how trivial the sign or how little the other person means to him.

While the first of these steps shows the patient the extent of his particular problem, the second impresses upon his mind the intensity of the forces behind it. Both arouse an interest in further scrutiny.

When it comes to examining the subjective value of a particular trend, the patient himself will often be eager to volunteer information. He may point out that his rebellion and defiance against authority or against anything resembling coercion were necessary and indeed lifesaving, since otherwise he would have been submerged by a dominating parent; that notions of superiority helped or still help to keep him going in the face of his lack of self-respect; that his detachment or his "don't-care" attitude protects him from being hurt. It is true that associations of this kind come forth in a spirit of defense, but they are also revealing. They tell us something about the reasons why the particular attitude was acquired in the first place, thereby showing us its historical value and giving us a better under-

standing of the patient's development. But over and beyond this, they lead the way to an understanding of the
present functions of the trend. From the standpoint of
therapy these are the functions of prime interest. No
neurotic trend or conflict is merely a relic from the
past—a habit, as it were, that once established keeps
persisting. We can be sure that it is determined by
stringent necessities within the existing character structure. The mere knowledge of why a neurotic peculiarity developed originally can only be of secondary value,
since what we must change are the forces that operate
at present.

For the most part, the subjective value of any neurotic position lies in its counterbalancing some other
neurotic tendency. A thorough comprehension of these
values, therefore, will provide an indication of how
to proceed in any particular instance. If, for example,
we are aware that a patient cannot relinquish his feeling
of omnipotence because it permits him to mistake his
potentialities for realities, his glorious projects for
actual accomplishments, we shall know that we must
examine the extent to which he lives in imagination.
And if he lets us see that he lives this way in order to
ensure himself against failure, our attention will be
directed toward the factors that lead him not only to
anticipate failure but to be in constant dread of it.

The most important therapeutic step is to bring the
patient to see the reverse side of the medal: the in-
capacitating effects of his neurotic drives and conflicts.
Some of this work will have been covered during the
preceding steps; but it is essential that the picture be
complete in all its detail. Only then will the patient

actually feel the need of changing. In view of the fact that every neurotic is driven to maintain the status quo, an incentive powerful enough to outweigh the retarding forces is required. Such an incentive, however, can come only from his desire for inner freedom, happiness, and growth, and from the realization that every neurotic difficulty stands in the way of its fulfillment. Thus if he tends toward derogatory self-criticism he must see how this dissipates his self-respect and leaves him without hope; how it makes him feel unwanted, compelling him to suffer abuse, which in turn causes him to be vindictive; how it paralyzes his incentive and ability to work; how, in order to keep from falling into the abyss of self-contempt, he is forced into defensive attitudes like self-aggrandizement, remoteness from himself, and feelings of unreality about himself, so perpetuating his neurosis.

Similarly, when a particular conflict has become visible during the analytical process, the patient must be made aware of its influence upon his life. In the case of a conflict between self-effacing tendencies and a need for triumph, all the cramping inhibitions inherent in inverted sadism must be understood. The patient must see how he responds to every self-effacing move with self-contempt, and with rage at the person before whom he cringes; and how, on the other hand, he responds to every attempt to triumph over someone with horror of himself and a fear of retaliation.

It sometimes happens that a patient, even when he becomes aware of the whole range of adverse consequences, shows no interest in overcoming the particular neurotic attitude. Instead, the problem seems to fade out of the picture. Almost imperceptibly he shoves it aside and nothing is gained. In view of the fact that he has seen all the harm he inflicts upon himself, his lack of response is remarkable. Nevertheless, unless the analyst is very astute in recognizing this kind of reaction, the patient's lack of interest may pass unnoticed. The patient takes up another subject, the analyst follows him, until they arrive again at a similar impasse. Only much later will the analyst become aware of the fact that the changes that have taken place in the patient are not commensurate with the amount of work done.

If the analyst knows that a reaction of this kind can occasionally be expected, he will ask himself what factors at work within the patient prevent him from accepting the fact that the particular attitude with its train of harmful consequences must be changed. There are usually a number of such factors, and they can only be tackled bit by bit. The patient may still be too paralyzed by hopelessness to consider the possibility of change. His drive to triumph over the analyst, to frustrate him, to let him make a fool of himself, may be stronger than his self-interest. His tendency to externalize may still be so great that in spite of his recognition of the consequences he cannot apply the insight to himself. His need to feel omnipotent may still be so strong that even though he sees the consequences as inevitable he makes a mental reservation that he will be able to get around them. His idealized image may still be so rigid that he cannot accept himself with any neurotic attitudes or conflicts. He will then merely rage against himself and feel that he ought to be able to master the particular difficulty simply because he is cognizant of it. It is important to be aware of these possibilities, because if the factors that choke the patient's incentive to change are overlooked, the analysis can easily degenerate into what Houston Peterson calls a "mania psychologica," a psychology for psychology's sake. Bringing the patient to accept himself under these circumstances constitutes a distinct gain. Even though nothing in the conflict itself has undergone change, he will have a profound sense of relief and will begin to show signs of wanting to disentangle the web in which he is caught. Once this favorable condition for work has been established, changes will soon begin to occur.

Needless to say, the above presentation is not meant to be a treatise on analytical technique. I have attempted to cover neither all the aggravating factors that operate during the process nor all the curative ones. I have not discussed, for instance, any of the difficulties or benefits that arise in connection with the patient's bringing all his defensive and offensive peculiarities into the relationship with the analyst—though this is an element of great significance. The steps I have described constitute merely the essential processes that must be gone through each time a new trend or conflict becomes visible. It is often impossible to proceed in the order named, since a problem may be inaccessible to the patient even when it has come into sharp focus. As we saw in the example concerning the arrogation of rights, one problem may merely disclose another which must be analyzed first. As long as every step is eventually covered, the order is of secondary importance.

The specific symptomatic changes that result from
analytical work naturally vary with the subject tackled.
A state of panic may subside when the patient recognizes his unconscious impotent rage and its background.
A depression may lift when he sees the dilemma in
which he was caught. But each piece of analysis well
done also brings about certain general changes in the
patient's attitude toward others and toward himself,
changes that occur regardless of the particular problem
that has been worked through. If we were to take such
dissimilar problems as an overemphasis on sex, a belief
that reality will accord with one's wishful thinking, and
a hypersensitivity to coercion, we would find that their
analysis affects the personality in much the same way.
No matter which of these difficulties is analyzed, hostility, helplessness, fear, and alienation from the self
and others will be diminished. Let us consider, for
example, how alienation from the self is lessened in
each of these instances. A person who overemphasizes
sex feels alive only in sexual experiences and fantasies;
his triumphs and defeats are confined within the sexual
sphere; the only asset he values in himself is his sexual
attractiveness. It is only when he understands this condition that he can start to become interested in other
aspects of living, and so retrieve himself. A person for
whom reality is bounded by the projects and plans of
his imagination has lost sight of himself as a functioning human being. He sees neither his limitations nor
his actual assets. Through analytical work he ceases to
mistake his potentialities for accomplishments; he is
able not only to face but to feel himself as he really is.
The person who is hypersensitive to coercion has be-

come oblivious to his own desires and beliefs, and feels that it is others who dominate and impose upon him. When this condition is analyzed, he begins to know what he really wants, and hence is able to strive toward his own goals.

In every analysis repressed hostility, regardless of its kind and source, will come to the fore and make the patient temporarily more irritable. But each time a neurotic attitude is abandoned, irrational hostility will be diminished. The patient will be less hostile when he sees his own share in the difficulty instead of externalizing, and when he becomes less vulnerable, less fearful, less dependent, less demanding, and so on.

Hostility is primarily allayed by a decrease in helplessness. The stronger a person becomes, the less he feels threatened by others. The accrual of strength stems from various sources. His center of gravity, which had been shifted to others, comes to rest within himself; he feels more active and starts to establish his own set of values. He will gradually have more energy available: the energy that had gone into repressing part of himself is released; he becomes less inhibited, less paralyzed by fears, self-contempt, and hopelessness. Instead of either blindly complying or fighting or venting sadistic impulses, he can give in on a rational basis and so becomes firmer.

Finally, although anxiety is temporarily stirred up by the undermining of established defenses, each step that is profitably taken is bound to diminish it, because the patient becomes less afraid of others and of himself.

The general result of these changes is an improvement in the patient's relations with others and with himself. He becomes less isolated; to the extent that he becomes stronger and less hostile, others gradually cease to be a menace to be fought, manipulated, or avoided. He can afford to have friendly feelings for them. His relations with himself improve as externalization is relinquished and self-contempt disappears.

If we examine the changes that take place during analysis we see that they apply to the very conditions that brought about the original conflicts. While in the course of a neurotic development all the stresses become more acute, therapy takes the opposite road. The attitudes that arose from the necessity of coping with the world in the face of helplessness, fear, hostility, and isolation become more and more meaningless and hence can be gradually dispensed with. Why, indeed, should anyone want to efface or sacrifice himself for persons he hates and who step on him if he has the capacity to meet others on an equal footing? Why should anyone have an insatiable desire for power and recognition if he feels secure within himself and can live and strive with others without the constant fear of being submerged? Why should anyone anxiously avoid involvement with others if he is able to love and is not afraid to fight?

To do this work takes time; the more entangled and the more barricaded a person is, the more time is required. That there should be a desire for brief analytical therapy is quite understandable. We should like to see more persons benefit from all that analysis has to offer, and we realize that some help is better than no help at all. Neuroses, it is true, vary greatly in severity, and mild neuroses can be helped in a comparatively short period. While some of the experiments in brief psychotherapy are promising, many, unfortunately, are based upon wishful thinking and are carried on with an ignorance of the powerful forces that operate in neurosis. In the case of severe neuroses I believe that the analytical procedure can be shortened only by so bettering our understanding of the neurotic character structure that less time will be wasted in groping for interpretations.

Fortunately analysis is not the only way to resolve inner conflicts. Life itself still remains a very effective therapist. Experience of any one of a number of kinds may be sufficiently telling to bring about personality changes. It may be the inspiring example of a truly great person; it may be a common tragedy which by bringing the neurotic in close touch with others takes him out of his egocentric isolation; it may be association with persons so congenial that manipulating or avoiding them appears less necessary. In other instances the consequences of neurotic behavior may be so drastic or of such frequent occurrence that they impress themselves on the neurotic's mind and make him less fearful and less rigid.

The therapy effected by life itself is not, however, within one's control. Neither hardships nor friendships nor religious experience can be arranged to meet the needs of the particular individual. Life as a therapist is ruthless; circumstances that are helpful to one neurotic may entirely crush another. And, as we have seen, the capacity of the neurotic to recognize the consequences of his neurotic behavior and to learn from them is highly limited. We could rather say that an analysis can be safely terminated if the patient has acquired this very capacity to learn from his experiences—that is, if he can examine his share in the difficulties that arise, understand it, and apply the insight to his life.

Knowledge of the role that conflicts play in neurosis and the realization that they can be resolved make it necessary to redefine the goals of analytical therapy. Although many neurotic disturbances belong in the medical sphere, it is not feasible to define the goals in medical terms. Since even psychosomatic illnesses are essentially an ultimate expression of conflicts within the personality, the goals of therapy must be defined in terms of personality.

Thus seen they encompass a number of aims. The patient must acquire the capacity to assume *responsibility* for himself, in the sense of feeling himself the active, responsible force in his life, capable of making decisions and of taking the consequences. With this goes an acceptance of responsibility toward others, a readiness to recognize obligations in whose value he believes, whether they relate to his children, parents, friends, employees, colleagues, community, or country.

Closely allied is the aim of achieving an *inner independence*—one as far removed from a mere defiance of the opinions and beliefs of others as from a mere adoption of them. This would mean primarily enabling the patient to establish his own hierarchy of values and to apply it to his actual living. In reference to others it would entail respect for their individuality and their rights, and would thus be the basis for a real mutuality. It would coincide with truly democratic ideals.

We could define the goals in terms of *spontaneity of*

feeling, an awareness and aliveness of feeling, whether in respect to love or hate, happiness or sadness, fear or desire. This would include a capacity for expression as well as for voluntary control. Because it is so vital, the capacity for love and friendship should be especially mentioned in this context; love that is neither parasitic dependence nor sadistic domination but, to quote Macmurray,[3] "a relationship . . . which has no purpose beyond itself; in which we associate because it is natural for human beings to share their experience; to understand one another, to find joy and satisfaction in living together; in expressing and revealing themselves to one another."

The most comprehensive formulation of therapeutic goals is the striving for *wholeheartedness:* to be without pretense, to be emotionally sincere, to be able to put the whole of oneself into one's feelings, one's work, one's beliefs. It can be approximated only to the extent that conflicts are resolved.

These goals are not arbitrary, nor are they valid goals of therapy simply because they coincide with the ideals that wise persons of all times have followed. But the coincidence is not accidental, for these are the elements upon which psychic health rests. We are justified in postulating these goals because they follow logically from a knowledge of the pathogenic factors in neurosis.

Our daring to name such high goals rests upon the belief that the human personality can change. It is not only the young child who is pliable. All of us retain the capacity to change, even to change in fundamental ways, as long as we live. This belief is supported by ex-

[3] John Macmurray, *op. cit.*

perience. Analysis is one of the most potent means of bringing about radical changes, and the better we understand the forces operating in neurosis the greater our chance of effecting desired change.

Neither the analyst nor the patient is likely wholly to attain these goals. They are ideals to strive for; their practical value lies in their giving us direction in our therapy and in our lives. If we are not clear about the meaning of ideals, we run the danger of replacing an old idealized image with a new one. We must be aware, too, that it does not lie within the power of the analyst to turn the patient into a flawless human being. He can only help him to become free to strive toward an approximation of these ideals. And this means giving him as well an opportunity to mature and develop.

Index

Academy of Medicine, 7

Adler, A., 99

Aggressive drives, uncovering, 58; and sadism, 210

Aggressive trends, 55, 63 ff; projection of, 126

Aggressive type, and anxiety, 64; attitudes, 69; efficiency of, 67; his "realism," 67; his need of exploitation, 65; inhibitions, 68; need for recognition, 70; throttling of feelings, 68; versus compliant type, 65, 66, 71

Alexander, Franz, 11, 99; "The Relation of Structural and Instinctual Conflicts," 38

Alienation from the self, 18, 111, 134, 144, 160

American Institute for Psychoanalysis, 7

Analysis, duration of, 239; errors in, 227; intuition in, 227; termination of, 241

Analytical technique, procedure in analysis, 228, 230 ff; sequence in analysis, 222; timing of interpretations, 223, 224; watchfulness of reactions, 235

Analytical therapy, aims and goals, 241, 242

Anxiety, 13, 41, 43, 64, 75; during analysis, 238; and sadism, 208, 209

Appel, Kenneth E. (and Edward A. Strecker), *Discovering Ourselves,* 116, 133

Arbitrary rightness, functions of, 137, 138

Armi, Anna Maria, 82

Arrogance, and idealized image, 96; neurotic, 167, 168

Artificial harmony, 131 ff; and rationalization, 135

Association for the Advancement of Psychoanalysis, 7

Associations, interpretations of, 225, 228, 232

Barrie, J. M., *Tommy and Grizel,* 111

Basic attitudes, 14

Basic conflict, 16, 18, 36, 37, 40, 47, 48, 71, 100; attempts at solution, 16, 131, 220; defenses, 135 ff; definition of, 37; Freud's opinion on, 38, 39; understanding of, 48, 222

Chekhov, Anton, *The Cherry Orchard,* 185.

Childhood, experiences of, 13, 45; exploring of, 128, 129; relative importance of, 213, 218

Claustrophobia, 78

Compartmentalization, 133, 134, 167

Books That Live

THE NORTON IMPRINT ON A BOOK
MEANS THAT IN THE PUBLISHER'S
ESTIMATION IT IS A BOOK NOT FOR A
SINGLE SEASON BUT FOR THE YEARS

W · W · NORTON & COMPANY · INC ·